The Diabetes Cookbook
for Electric Pressure Cookers

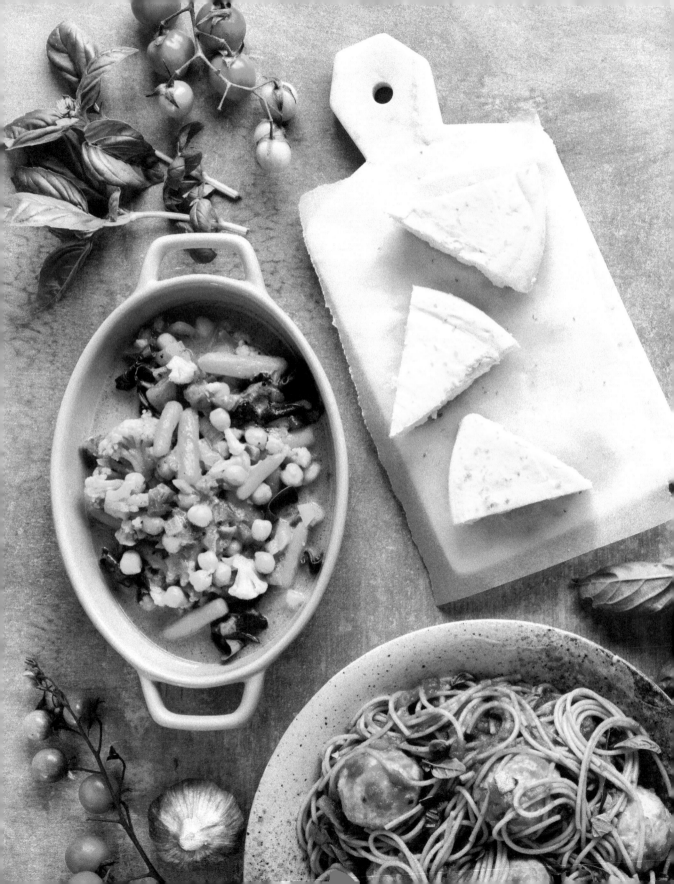

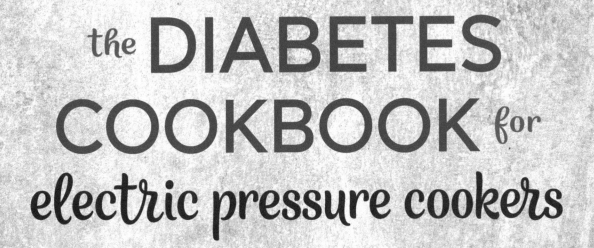

the DIABETES COOKBOOK for electric pressure cookers

Instant Healthy Meals for Managing Diabetes

SHELBY KINNAIRD
SIMONE HAROUNIAN, MS, RD, CDN, CDE

Photography by Nadine Greeff

R

ROCKRIDGE
PRESS

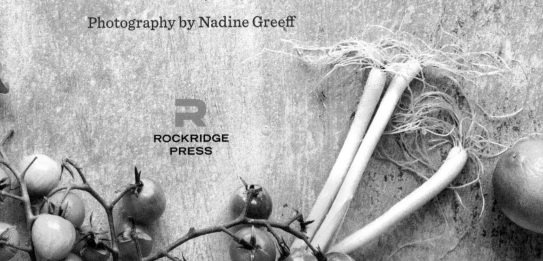

For general information on our other products and services or to obtain technical support, please contact our Customer Care Department within the United States at (866) 744-2665, or outside the United States at (510) 253-0500.

Rockridge Press publishes its books in a variety of electronic and print formats. Some content that appears in print may not be available in electronic books, and vice versa.

TRADEMARKS: Rockridge Press and the Rockridge Press logo are trademarks or registered trademarks of Callisto Media Inc. and/or its affiliates, in the United States and other countries, and may not be used without written permission. All other trademarks are the property of their respective owners. Rockridge Press is not associated with any product or vendor mentioned in this book.

Interior and Cover Designer: Liz Cosgrove
Photo Art Director: Sue Smith
Editor: Kim Suarez
Production Editor: Andrew Yackira
Photography © Nadine Greeff, 2019.
Author photo (Shelby) courtesy A Click in Time Photography.

ISBN: Print 978-1-64152-288-5
eBook 978-1-64152-289-2

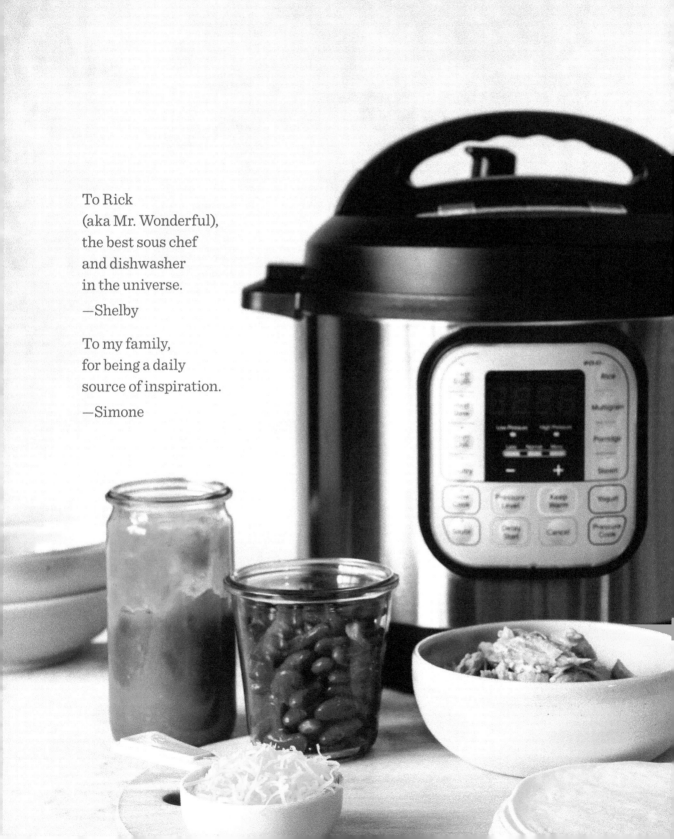

To Rick
(aka Mr. Wonderful),
the best sous chef
and dishwasher
in the universe.

—Shelby

To my family,
for being a daily
source of inspiration.

—Simone

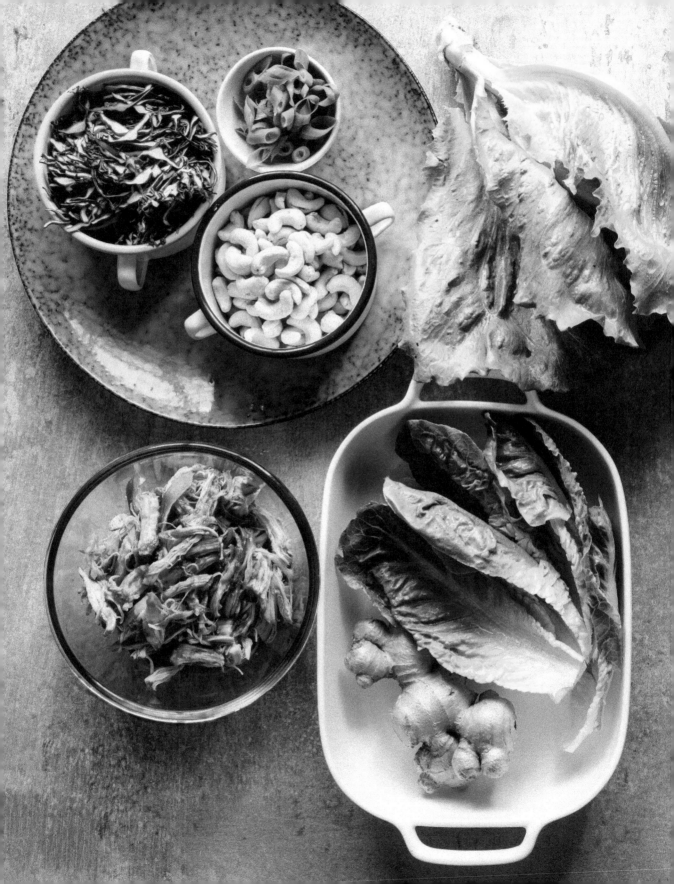

Contents

Introduction

There are many reasons you may be reading this book right now. Perhaps one (or more) of these statements describe you:

- I have diabetes, and I don't know what to eat.

- I don't have time to cook healthy meals.

- I bought an electric pressure cooker (EPC) on sale, but it's still in the box.

- I take care of someone who has diabetes, and I don't know what to feed them.

- I'm sick of cooking the same meals over and over.

- I'm tired of making a "healthy" meal for myself and a second meal for the rest of my family.

- I want healthy, delicious recipes that are easy to prepare.

- I hate cooking because it messes up so many pots and pans.

For those who can identify with any of the above, this book can help you make quick and easy, diabetes-friendly meals in the EPC that your entire family will love. If you don't have diabetes but just like to eat healthy, you'll find plenty here to please your palate, too. If you are eating more meatless meals, there's an entire chapter devoted to those. Plus, there are many gluten-free, vegan, and low-sodium recipes spread throughout the book. I've even included some desserts if you're in the mood to splurge.

When I was a kid, my mom cooked in a stovetop pressure cooker at least once a week. I remember hearing the steamy jiggle of the regulator on top, then watching Mom carry

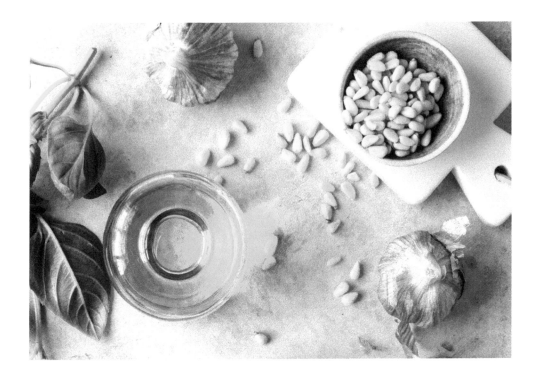

the pot to the sink to run water over it before daring to lift off the cover. Usually, the most amazing-smelling chicken would be inside. Even though I've always liked to cook, I never learned how to use one of those stovetop units.

Once I discovered the electric, multi-function pressure cookers, I was all in. I learned you can prepare a whole chicken or bone-in turkey breast easily, plus do a lot of other things like cook dried beans in about an hour (no soaking required), steam corn on the cob, "hard-boil" eggs that are easy to peel, and make cheesecake without the top cracking. You can also sauté right in the pot, unlike most slow cookers, which require you to brown things on the stove, then transfer them to the cooker.

If you're the type of person who plans one or two meal prep days a week, you'll love using an EPC. It's so easy to make nutrient-rich soups or stews in large quantities quickly and freeze premeasured portions. You can also cook beans and chickpeas and make your own bone broth to store for later use.

If you're not much of a planner, you'll find the EPC works for you as well. If you forget to thaw meat for dinner, you can throw it into the pot still frozen. It may seem like it is all too good to be true, but really, you can prepare delicious diabetes-friendly meals that come together quickly and easily using your EPC. Welcome to the world of pressure cooking!

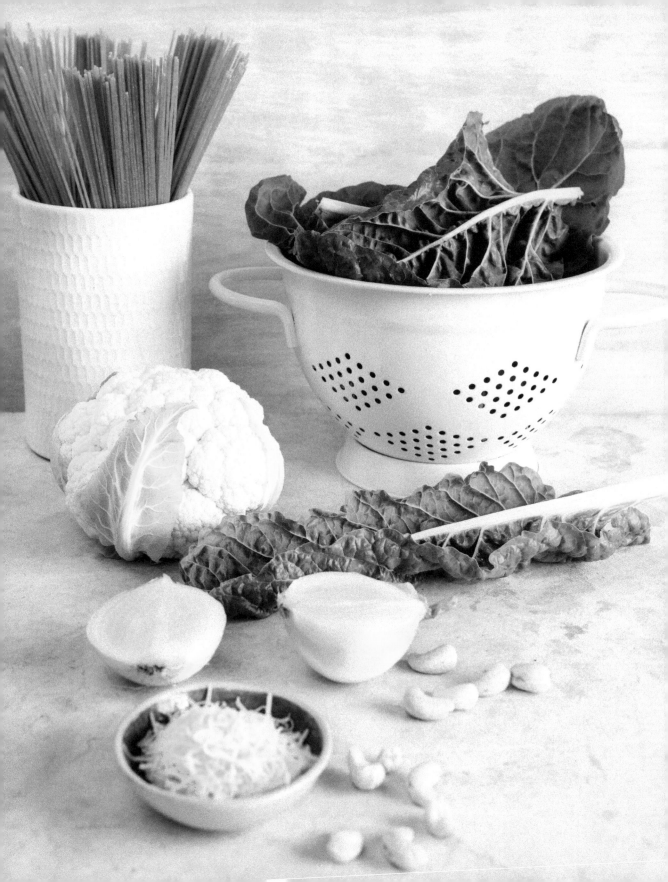

1

Take the Pressure Off of Managing Diabetes

For me, by far, the most important aspect of diabetes management over the years has been eating meals at home. When I eat food I've prepared myself, I'm able to keep my blood sugar in range and my weight steady. When I eat more restaurant meals, that picture changes. When I get busy, I feel I have no time to cook, and cooking something that should be "easy" on the stovetop is far from it on those stressful days.

Enter the EPC. Cooking with an EPC requires minimal planning, and clean-up is a breeze. You can usually create something tasty from ingredients already in your pantry and refrigerator. You can set the table and unload the dishwasher while your meal cooks. You can even cook meat without defrosting it first.

Managing your diabetes just got a whole lot easier.

—Shelby

The Benefits of the EPC

The key to a healthy diet for managing diabetes is portion control, but it is just as important to be aware of the types of foods you eat. Here are a few guidelines for eating healthfully for diabetes, along with a few ways in which the EPC can help make cooking those foods easier and more convenient.

Be mindful of portion sizes.

Portion control is a challenge for most of us. It is difficult to eat the right amount of food when hunger is driving our decision-making. The EPC is great for solving this challenge. One of the most convenient features of the EPC is the ability to prepare large batches of meals and side dishes ahead of time. You can then pre-portion the food, and later on, when it is time to eat, there is no second-guessing the proper portion sizes.

Choose foods as close to nature as possible.

When you choose foods as close to nature as possible, you increase your intake of good-for-you nutrients such as vitamins, minerals, fiber, and antioxidants, all of which protect your body. Once these foods are cooked, they can lose some of their nutritional value. Nutrients often leach out of the food and into the cooking water. The EPC prepares foods with high heat, minimal water, and in a shorter duration. This method optimizes the nutritional content by retaining more vitamins and minerals than any other cooking method.

Eat fewer refined carbohydrates and more whole grains.

Refined carbohydrates such as white pasta and white rice should be limited or even eliminated from your diet, since they can have an immediate impact on your blood sugar levels. The good news is, choosing whole grain counterparts like whole wheat pasta and brown rice can be enjoyed in moderation. These foods take longer to cook because of their higher fiber content. The EPC allows you to cook whole grains such as farro, barley, and black rice quickly and in large servings to freeze as leftovers.

Choose lean protein instead of higher fat protein.

It is recommended to choose leaner cuts of meat to keep your heart healthy, but that often comes at the sacrifice of flavor. The EPC uses water with high-pressure heat. This technique seals in moisture and produces a more tender and juicier meat—without all the harmful fat. Seasoning lean proteins with herbs and spices, as you'll see in the recipes in this book, can intensify flavors so you won't be missing any of that fat.

🗃 Diabetes-Friendly Vegetables for the EPC

The EPC is a valuable gadget to help you incorporate more vegetables in your diet. While vegetables offer enormous health benefits by providing fiber, vitamins, minerals, and antioxidants, it must be stressed that not all vegetables are considered equal when monitoring your carbohydrate intake.

Vegetables with less than 5 grams of carbohydrates per serving, or non-starchy vegetables, can be consumed in almost unlimited quantities, as they don't have a significant impact on increasing your blood sugar levels. This is great news, since these vegetables are low in calories, full of water, and keep you full for longer, which can aid in weight loss.

Vegetables with more than 10 grams of carbohydrates per serving, or starchy vegetables, must be consumed in moderation, as they can cause blood sugar levels to spike at a quick rate. While they don't need to be eliminated from your diet, since they still offer plenty of nutrients, you must be cautious of portion size to prevent a significant impact on your blood sugar. Although it varies by vegetable, a general recommendation is that the total carbohydrate portion of your meal should be no larger than the size of your fist.

Below are two lists of EPC-friendly vegetables: non-starchy carbs on the left and starchy carbs on the right. Don't forget to mind the portion size!

NON-STARCHY VEGETABLES		STARCHY VEGETABLES
Asparagus	Leeks	Acorn squash
Beets	Mushrooms	Butternut squash
Broccoli	Okra	Corn
Brussels sprouts	Onions	Green peas
Cabbage	Pea pods	Lima beans
Carrots	Peppers	Parsnips
Cauliflower	Radishes	Plantains
Celery	Rutabaga	Potatoes
Eggplant	Spaghetti squash	Pumpkin
Green beans	Summer squash (zucchini, yellow squash)	Yams or sweet potatoes
Greens	Swiss chard	
Jicama	Tomatoes	
Kohlrabi	Turnips	

Cut caloric intake to help with weight loss.

Consuming fewer calories throughout the day can help with weight loss and blood glucose management. The EPC can make soups, chili, and vegetable dishes with little to no oil, giving you lots of options for low-calorie meals and side dishes.

Incorporate more plant-based foods.

Your choices for preparing vegetables are endless, due to the many different functions of the EPC. You can use the recipes in this book to experiment and find the foods and flavors that appeal to you most. As an example, the EPC makes it quicker and easier to cook beans and legumes. And as an added bonus, it makes them much easier to digest, too!

EPC Meal Planning and the Plate Method

You probably hear a lot about *what* you should eat: vegetables, fruits, whole grains, beans and legumes, lean protein, low-fat dairy, and plant-based oils. But what is not emphasized enough is *how much* of these foods you should consume. It can be confusing, especially when you are influenced by the oversized portions in restaurants and television commercials. Large portions of anything (even healthy food) can lead to overeating, high blood sugar, and eventually unwanted weight gain. The Plate Method is one tool you can use on your own to build a healthy meal.

If you are aware of the proper portion sizes for the various food groups, it becomes much easier to make sure your meals are balanced, include a variety of nutrients, and satisfy your hunger. Each person has individualized recommendations for nutrients they require to make sure their body works optimally, but you must meet with a registered dietitian to determine this.

The Plate Method

Imagine an empty dinner plate (approximately nine inches in diameter) right in front of you. Now, imagine a line dividing the plate in half. Divide one half of the plate again, keeping the other half intact. You are now looking at a plate that has three sections—one section is half the plate, and the other two sections are a quarter of the plate.

- **The half of your plate is for non-starchy vegetables.** Load this area up! Not only do these vegetables keep you fuller for longer, but they can also help keep your blood sugar from spiking high too quickly and help prevent cravings. When putting your meal together, make sure to choose at least two vegetables with different colors. If you have a variety of colors on your plate, you will be getting a variety of vitamins, minerals, and antioxidants.

- **The next quarter of your plate is for lean protein.** Protein includes foods like poultry, eggs, red meat, fish, shellfish, or soy products. Protein doesn't have an immediate impact on your blood sugar, but choosing protein high in animal fat can negatively affect your heart. When choosing meats, keep it lean and go for white meat poultry without the skin or lean cuts of red meat (flank steak, top loin, sirloin, tenderloin, or 90-percent lean ground beef). Fish is an excellent source of protein that can also provide omega-3 fatty acids, which studies show are beneficial for heart health. Make sure to incorporate fish in your diet at least twice a week to reap the benefits.

- **The last quarter of your plate is for starch or grains.** Starches include starchy vegetables like corn, peas, some squash, or potatoes. Grains include bread, rice, pasta, and ancient grains like quinoa or farro. Since beans are made of both protein and starch, they go here. This section of your plate can have an immediate impact on your blood sugar, so it's best to keep this portion to an amount that is no larger than a tight fist. When choosing grains, go with whole wheat or whole grain options such as whole wheat pasta and brown rice. These options have more fiber than the white varieties, and they won't raise blood sugar levels quite as high.

The keys to implementing the Plate Method are meal planning and preparing ahead of time. You can also use portion-control dinnerware from companies like Livliga® to make things easier. If you plan out what you are going to eat throughout the week, with careful attention to vegetables, protein, and starches/grains, you will have options in front of you to build a healthy plate.

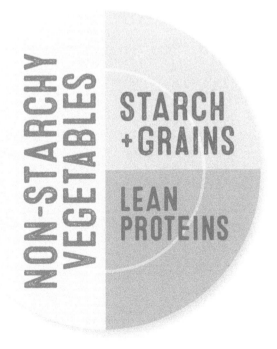

NON-STARCHY VEGETABLES

STARCH +GRAINS

LEAN PROTEINS

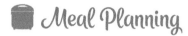 # Meal Planning

Meal planning is essential for healthy eating. The EPC can make thinking ahead even more of a breeze! By preplanning and using the make-ahead steps in the recipes in this book, you can put together a meal plan that's healthy, delicious, and—most importantly—convenient. Here is a sample week's menu. Each meal is balanced with protein and fiber to keep you satisfied. The lunches are

	SUNDAY	MONDAY	TUESDAY
Breakfast	Gouda Egg Casserole with Canadian Bacon (page 18) Fresh berries	Tropical Steel Cut Oats (page 23) ¼ cup pumpkin or sunflower seeds	Poached Eggs (page 22) Slice of 100% whole wheat bread Sautéed spinach Tomato slices
Lunch	Buttercup Squash Soup (page 37) Tossed salad with ¼ cup walnuts	Beef in lettuce wraps from Mary's Sunday Pot Roast leftovers Leftover Buttercup Squash Soup	Lentils with Carrots (page 61) with leftover turkey from Herbed Whole Turkey Breast
Dinner	Mary's Sunday Pot Roast (page 92) Steamed broccoli	Herbed Whole Turkey Breast (page 79) Sautéed carrots and string beans	Pork Carnitas (page 94) Corn tortilla (or lettuce wrap) Salsa verde Avocado
Do-Ahead Prep	Prepare lettuce cups Prep carrots and string beans for dinner	Cook Lentils with Carrots with the leftover turkey breast for lunch Zest and juice orange and lime for Carnitas	Make Posole with leftover pork for lunch Make salad for lunch Cut vegetables in quarters to roast for dinner

designed to use leftovers and/or repurpose your dinner from the night before. The "Do-Ahead Prep" section outlines steps that will make cooking the next day effortless. Eating healthy is now as easy as pressing the Pressure Cook button on your EPC!

WEDNESDAY	THURSDAY	FRIDAY	SATURDAY
Blueberry Oat Mini Muffin (page 24) ¼ cup almonds	Smoked Salmon and Asparagus Quiche Cups (page 19) Fresh melon	Breakfast Farro with Berries and Walnuts (page 25)	Shakshuka with Swiss Chard (page 20)
4-Ingredient Carnitas Posole (page 45) (leftovers from Pork Carnitas) Tossed salad	Shredded chicken from Smoky Whole Chicken leftovers Sautéed asparagus, zucchini, cauliflower	Minestrone with Red Beans, Zucchini, and Spinach leftovers	Black Bean Soup with Lime-Yogurt Drizzle (page 41)
Smoky Whole Chicken (page 70) Roasted veggies: Brussels sprouts, beets	Minestrone with Red Beans, Zucchini, and Spinach (page 54)	Chicken Salsa Verde with Pumpkin (page 74) made with leftovers from Smoky Whole Chicken (page 70)	Cauliflower Chickpea Curry (page 60)
Prepare asparagus and onion for Quiche Sauté asparagus, zucchini, cauliflower for lunch	Cook chickpeas for Curry on Saturday	Prepare onion for Shakshuka and Curry	

The Diabetes-Friendly Kitchen

For the EPC to make your life easier, you'll need to stock your pantry, refrigerator, and freezer with some essentials. At a minimum, you'll want salt and pepper, cooking oil, spices, onions, and garlic. I keep a few pots of fresh herbs, like rosemary, thyme, parsley, and chives, but I also have a jar of chopped garlic and a tube of minced ginger in my refrigerator when I'm pressed for time. A wide variety of fruits, vegetables, beans, and whole grains can help you whip up healthy meals quickly in your EPC.

The Pantry

SPICES

- **Bay leaves.** You may think bay leaves are optional when you see them in a list of ingredients, but don't skip them. They add subtle background flavors to soups and stews. I like the Turkish ones from Penzeys Spices.

- **Chili powder.** Keep different varieties of chili powder in your spice rack. At any given time, I'll have chipotle, ancho, and regular blends that range from mild to hot.

- **Cinnamon.** If you want to add a touch of sweetness to a dish without any carbs, try ground cinnamon. It works in both sweet and savory recipes. When I'm in the mood for extra pizzazz, I use Moxy Kitchen's Spicy Cinnamon Mix.

- **Nutmeg.** Like cinnamon, nutmeg works in both sweet and savory dishes. Buy some ground nutmeg or blends like apple pie spice or pumpkin pie spice that include it. Also purchase whole nutmeg and a Microplane to use it freshly grated.

- **Pepper.** Everyone needs an arsenal of pepper choices. I frequently use freshly ground black pepper, a black and red pepper blend from McCormick called Hot Shot!, garlic pepper, cayenne pepper, and white pepper (when I don't want black specks in my dish).

- **Spice blends.** Combination spices like Italian seasoning and herbes de Provence can save you some time and perk up a dish. If a recipe calls for dried basil, rosemary, thyme, and oregano, use Italian seasoning instead. If it calls for dried thyme, oregano, marjoram, rosemary, and savory, use herbes de Provence.

LEGUMES

- **Beans.** Keep beans around in both dried and canned forms. A great source of fiber and vitamins, beans may help lower cholesterol and reduce the spike in blood sugar that occurs after a meal. See Salt-Free No-Soak Beans (page 64) for information about cooking dried beans like black beans, pinto beans, and navy beans.

- **Chickpeas.** Also known as garbanzo beans, chickpeas are a great source of plant-based protein, folate, and fiber. Small studies have shown that chickpeas may decrease blood glucose levels, improve gut health, and lower blood cholesterol. Keep a few cans on hand, but also try cooking them yourself: see Salt-Free Chickpeas (page 58).

- **Lentils.** Brown lentils are sturdy and hold up well in soup. This is what you get when you buy generically labeled "lentils." Green lentils (Puy) are associated with French cooking and are used in lentil-based salads and side dishes. Red and yellow lentils are delicate, cook quickly, and are great for thickening soup and chili. Black (beluga) lentils look like caviar and are quite firm when cooked.

GRAINS

- **Barley.** A puffy, chewy, high-fiber whole grain, barley is best known for its starring role in soups. It's also great for breakfast, as a side, and in sweeter dishes.

- **Farro.** Similar to barley in texture, farro is a whole wheat grain that's packed with fiber, antioxidants, vitamins, and minerals.

- **Grits/polenta.** Grits and polenta are made from ground corn. They work well for breakfast or in savory dishes.

- **Rice.** Brown and black rice are higher in fiber and protein than white rice but have longer cooking times, making them perfect for the EPC. Wild rice, technically a grass, offers many nutrients, including zinc and magnesium.

- **Steel cut oats.** Also known as Irish oats, steel cut oats are huskless whole grain oat kernels that have been cut into smaller pieces with a steel blade. They are loaded with both soluble and insoluble fiber and take longer to cook than other types of oats, which makes them a good fit for the EPC.

PACKAGED, BOTTLED, CANNED

- **Avocado oil.** In general, olive oil is my fat of choice, but when sautéing in the EPC, I mainly use avocado oil because it has a higher smoke point. In sauté mode, the EPC can reach temperatures of 338°F (170°C), and the smoke point of extra virgin olive oil is 320°F (160°C). The smoke point of avocado oil is 520°F (271°C). Avocado oil isn't cheap, however. Less expensive alternatives include canola oil and peanut oil.

- **Broth.** Using broth or stock instead of water adds so much flavor to a dish. Keep lots of chicken stock and vegetable broth in the pantry. I prefer cartons to cans.

- **Sauces.** Quick meals using the EPC are easy when you have bottled sauces like salsa, salsa verde, pasta sauce, Worcestershire sauce, and soy sauce/tamari on hand. Pick the brands that are lowest in sodium and carbs.

- **Tomatoes.** Many of the recipes in this book feature tomatoes. Keep several options, like fire-roasted, diced, chopped, crushed, and tomatoes with green chilies, in your pantry. I prefer tomatoes stored in cartons to those stored in cans. Look for brands where the only ingredient is tomatoes.

- **Vinegars.** A quick shot of vinegar can add punch to a dish. You'll want apple cider vinegar, white wine vinegar, and a sweeter balsamic vinegar available as options.

The Fridge

- **Citrus fruit.** Keep a supply of lemons, limes, and oranges handy. You won't cook with them per se, but a squeeze of fresh citrus juice or a sprinkle of zest after cooking will really brighten a dish.

- **Eggs.** Many of the breakfast dishes in this book feature eggs, which cook beautifully in the EPC.

- **Leafy greens.** Always keep leafy greens in your refrigerator. You can make a quick side salad or stir some into a soup or stew for an extra boost of nutrition.

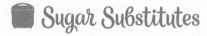 Sugar Substitutes

I honestly don't use many sugar substitutes. If I want to add sweetness to a dish, it's usually a little bit of honey or pure maple syrup. Here are sugar substitutes you may want to consider if you prefer lower-carb alternatives:

Monk fruit extract: Also known as *luo han guo* extract, monk fruit extract comes from an Asian gourd. This sugar substitute is heat stable, so it can be used in cooked or uncooked foods. For cooked or baked foods, substitute monk fruit extract for half of the sugar. For example, if the recipe calls for 1 cup of sugar, use ½ cup of monk fruit extract. In uncooked foods (e.g. to sweeten coffee), use a one-to-one substitution. Popular brands include Monk Fruit in the Raw® and PureLo®.

Stevia: Whole-leaf stevia is made from the dried leaves of the stevia plant, a completely natural sweetener. Refined, stevia-based sweeteners are processed, however. Whole-leaf stevia is not suitable for baking. Stevia-based sweeteners are available in powdered or liquid form: 1 teaspoon of either is equivalent to 1 cup of sugar. Popular brands include Truvia®, Pure Via™, and SweetLeaf Stevia®. Note that some with hay fever are sensitive to stevia, so use caution.

Swerve™: Favored by low-carb bakers because it measures cup for cup like sugar, Swerve is a combination of erythritol (a sugar alcohol), oligosaccharides (inulin), and "natural flavors." One teaspoon of Swerve contains 5 grams of carbohydrates, but the body does not metabolize these carbs and they have no impact on blood sugar. Three types of Swerve are available: one is granulated and similar to white table sugar, one is powdered and similar to confectioners' sugar, and the newest is brown and can be used as a substitute for light brown sugar.

- **Parmesan cheese.** I like to serve many dishes with a sprinkle of freshly grated Parmesan or Parmigiano-Reggiano cheese.

- **Vegetables.** Many recipes start out with *mirepoix*, the French term for a mixture of onions, celery, and carrots to add a flavor base. In Louisiana-style cooking, the mixture is known as "the Trinity," made of onions, celery, and bell pepper. Keep all of these vegetables on hand. On a food prep day, chop a big batch of onions and keep them in the fridge for easy access during the work week. A food processor works well for this task.

The Freezer

- **Fruit.** Frozen fruits work in so many dishes in the EPC. At a minimum, you'll want peaches, mango chunks, and berries.

- **Homemade broth.** Make Chicken Bone Broth (page 117) and Vegetable Broth (page 116) and store them in the freezer. When you make your own broth, which is so easy in the EPC, it will be more flavorful and you can control the amount of sodium.

- **Meat.** Stock up on lean cuts of beef and pork when they are on sale, and freeze them. If you plan to cook roasts frozen, cut them into smaller pieces before freezing.

- **Poultry.** Whole chickens are easy to cook in the EPC, as are bone-in breasts and boneless thighs. You can also cook boneless breasts, but you have to be careful, as they tend to dry out. Small turkey breasts and turkey tenderloins work well, too.

- **Vegetables.** Longer-cooking, more substantial vegetables like carrots, cauliflower, and winter squash work well in the EPC. Look for frozen brands that don't have added ingredients or sauces.

FAQs

Cooking with an EPC may very well change your life. Meals are quick and easy to prepare, and cleaning up is a breeze. Yet, the whole pressure cooking thing is still scary to many folks. Here are answers to some basic questions that will have you feeling confident with your EPC in no time.

Will my pressure cooker explode?

Most modern EPCs have built-in safety features that make an explosion highly unlikely. Yes, pressure will build up in the pot, but as long as you follow your manufacturer's directions for releasing the pressure before opening the pot, you'll be fine.

Why won't my EPC come to pressure?

You could have forgotten the sealing ring or not properly sealed it. You may have set the pressure release valve to venting instead of sealing. You may not have added enough liquid to the pot. Your float valve (pin) could be stuck.

What is the best way to clean my EPC?

Wash the inner pot in warm, soapy water or in the dishwasher after each use. For stubborn stains, I like to use Bar Keepers Friend (silver container). The lid should be rinsed after each use. If any food is stuck to the lid or the float valve, wash it off by hand using warm, soapy water. Periodically, remove the sealing ring and soak it in warm water with a little baking soda to remove odors. Wipe down the outside of the EPC and use a small foam paintbrush to make sure the rim stays clear of debris and liquid.

What is the difference between quick release and natural release?

Quick pressure release is when you release the pressure manually by moving the pressure release valve from sealing to venting. I use a long wooden spoon to do this, so my hand is nowhere near the steam. Once the pin drops, you can safely open the lid. Natural pressure release is when you allow the pot to sit after cooking is complete until the pressure is released and the pin drops on its own. Some recipes call for natural release for a certain amount of time and then a quick release of any remaining pressure.

Will food brown nicely?

Unlike most slow cookers, EPCs have sauté functions that allow you to brown foods before pressure cooking begins. Food will not get as brown as it does in the oven or on the stovetop, but it will be browner than it gets in a slow cooker.

Do I have to put water in the pot?

Pressure cooking involves steam, and generating steam requires liquid. Your liquid doesn't have to be water, but it should be thin like broth. Cooking foods that absorb a lot of liquid (e.g., beans) will require more liquid, while foods that release water (e.g., non-starchy vegetables) may require less. If you cook something in a pan inside your EPC's pot, you will need to put water in the bottom and place the pan on the wire rack or on a trivet. Make sure you know the minimum amount of liquid required for your particular EPC to come to pressure.

What accessories do I need to buy?

You don't *need* to buy any accessories, but you may *want* to. I frequently use a 7-inch springform pan, a 6-inch cake pan, an egg rack, a silicone egg bite mold, and 4-inch ramekins. An immersion blender also allows you to purée right in the pot. You can do quite a lot, however, simply with the wire rack that comes with the EPC.

I see steam all around the EPC's lid. Is that normal?

This probably means your sealing ring is missing. Move the pressure release valve from sealing to venting and wait for the pin to drop, then open the lid, let it cool, insert the sealing ring, and start over.

Whenever I cook something in the EPC, it smells like the last thing I cooked. How can I avoid this?

Smells often get trapped in the sealing ring. Remove the ring and soak it in a warm water–baking soda solution. You can also purchase additional rings that are fairly inexpensive. You may want to designate certain rings for heavily spiced dishes and others for milder foods, or one color for savory and another for sweet.

Why am I getting a burn notice?

If food starts to scorch at the bottom of the pot, you may see a burn notice indicator. There are several reasons this could happen:

- You don't have enough liquid in the pot.

- Your pot isn't properly sealed, and steam is leaking. The sealing ring may be missing or installed improperly. Your release valve may be set to venting instead of sealing.

- Food may have gotten stuck to the bottom, or the pot may have been too hot after you finished sautéing.

- You may be using an EPC that's a different size than the one in which the recipe was tested.

If I double the amount of ingredients, do I double the cooking time?

No. The EPC will take longer to come to pressure, but the cooking time should be the same.

Can I cook food that's frozen without defrosting it first?

Yes. Foods that have been frozen in a single layer or smaller pieces will work better than large chunks. If you plan to cook frozen roasts, cut them into smaller pieces before freezing. When you cook frozen foods, note that the EPC will take much longer to come to pressure than it would normally.

About the Recipes

All the recipes in this book were tested in a 6-quart Instant Pot Duo Plus. Adjustments may need to be made for other EPCs. In fact, when I was testing recipes for this book, I used two different EPCs (same model) and found differences in timings when using the Sauté setting. You'll need to get to know your own EPC in the same way you always need to get to know your oven.

For all the recipes here, Sauté means Sauté/Normal. A recipe requiring a higher or lower sauté temperature will be indicated by Sauté/More or Sauté/Less.

To make cooking as easy and streamlined as possible, for each recipe, you'll find a realistic *estimate* of how long it will take to make the dish, including prep time, cook time, the time it takes for pressure to build in the EPC, and total time.

Be sure to check out the labels on each recipe, too. These can help you determine if a recipe is appropriate for your nutritional circumstances or diet. The labels used include 20-Minutes-or-Less Prep, Vegan, Gluten Free, Family Friendly, Low Carb, Low Sodium, and Sugar Free. Dishes labeled "low carb" have less than 10g of carbohydrates per serving, those labeled "low sodium" contain 140mg or less of sodium per serving, those labeled "sugar free" contain less than .5g of sugar per serving, and those labeled "family friendly" contain 4 or more servings.

In each recipe, we have provided tips to make cooking and meal planning even easier. Make-ahead, Leftover, Repurpose, and Substitution tips will help make cooking and planning a breeze.

Finally, all of the recipes include nutritional information, so you can make the best decisions for your diabetes management.

Now, on to the recipes.

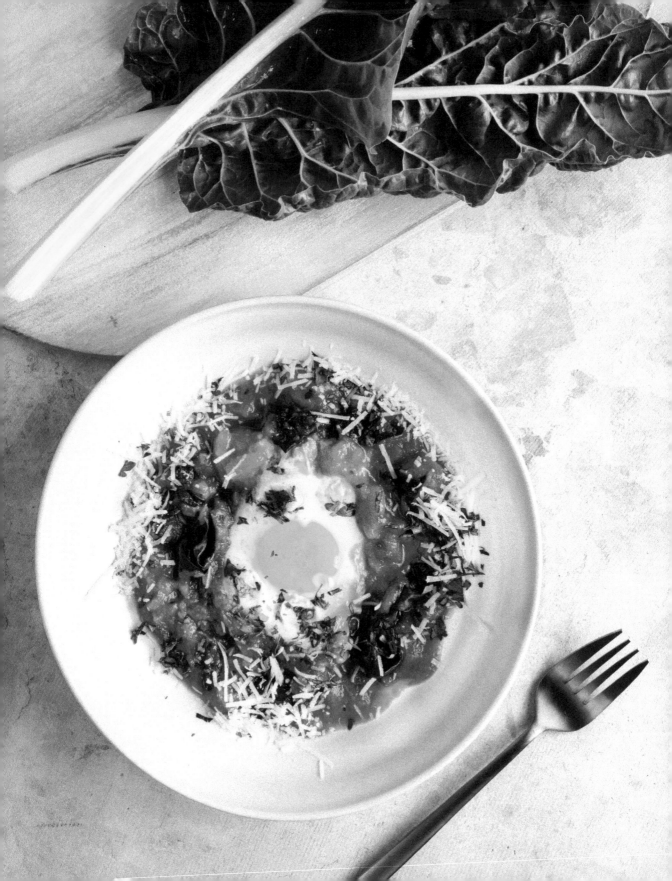

2

Breakfasts

PREP TIME:
12 minutes

COOK SETTING:
High

**PRESSURE-UP
TIME:** 7 minutes

COOK TIME:
20 minutes

RELEASE: Quick

TOTAL TIME:
45 minutes

**SPECIAL
EQUIPMENT:**
6-inch cake pan

20-MINUTES-OR-
LESS PREP

LOW CARB

FAMILY FRIENDLY

PER SERVING:
Calories: 247;
Total Fat: 15g; Protein: 20g;
Carbohydrates: 8g;
Sugars: 1g; Fiber: 1g;
Sodium: 717mg

Gouda Egg Casserole with Canadian Bacon

SERVES 4 (8G CARBS PER SERVING)

Breakfast on Christmas morning in our family usually involves a sausage and egg casserole featuring cheddar cheese. It's not the healthiest of options, but once a year I figure it's okay. Here, I've swapped Canadian bacon for the sausage and smoked Gouda for the cheddar to make a smaller casserole that cooks perfectly in an EPC. This version did get Mom and Dad's seal of approval.

Nonstick cooking spray

1 slice whole grain bread, toasted

½ cup shredded smoked
   Gouda cheese

3 slices Canadian bacon, chopped

6 large eggs

¼ cup half-and-half

¼ teaspoon kosher salt

¼ teaspoon freshly ground
   black pepper

¼ teaspoon dry mustard

1. Spray a 6-inch cake pan with cooking spray, or if the pan is nonstick, skip this step. If you don't have a 6-inch cake pan, any bowl or pan that fits inside your pressure cooker should work.

2. Crumble the toast into the bottom of the pan. Sprinkle with the cheese and Canadian bacon.

3. In a medium bowl, whisk together the eggs, half-and-half, salt, pepper, and dry mustard.

4. Pour the egg mixture into the pan. Loosely cover the pan with aluminum foil.

5. Pour 1½ cups water into the electric pressure cooker and insert a wire rack or trivet. Place the covered pan on top of the rack.

6. Close and lock the lid of the pressure cooker. Set the valve to sealing.

7. Cook on high pressure for 20 minutes.

8. When the cooking is complete, hit Cancel and quick release the pressure.

9. Once the pin drops, unlock and remove the lid.

10. Carefully transfer the pan from the pressure cooker to a cooling rack and let it sit for 5 minutes.

11. Cut into 4 wedges and serve.

Leftover tip: Reheat this casserole in the microwave for a perfectly portable breakfast. Be sure to remove it from the cake pan first and place it on a microwave-safe plate.

Smoked Salmon and Asparagus Quiche Cups

SERVES 2 (3G CARBS PER SERVING)

I read somewhere that raw vegetables shouldn't be included in EPC-cooked quiche because it messes up the texture. Stubbornly, I set out to prove this theory wrong. Here, both the onion and asparagus are added raw—and the texture is fine, thank you very much. I use white pepper because I think it looks nicer not to see dark specks in my quiche, but you can certainly use black pepper if that's what you have on hand.

Nonstick cooking spray

4 asparagus spears, cut into
½-inch pieces

2 tablespoons finely chopped onion

3 ounces smoked salmon (skinless and boneless), chopped

3 large eggs

2 tablespoons 2% milk

¼ teaspoon dried dill

Pinch ground white pepper

1. Pour 1½ cups of water into the electric pressure cooker and insert a wire rack or trivet.
2. Lightly spray the bottom and sides of the ramekins with nonstick cooking spray. Divide the asparagus, onion, and salmon between the ramekins.
3. In a measuring cup with a spout, whisk together the eggs, milk, dill, and white pepper. Pour half of the egg mixture into each ramekin. Loosely cover the ramekins with aluminum foil.
4. Carefully place the ramekins inside the pot on the rack.
5. Close and lock the lid of the pressure cooker. Set the valve to sealing.
6. Cook on high pressure for 15 minutes.
7. When the cooking is complete, hit Cancel and quick release the pressure.
8. Once the pin drops, unlock and remove the lid.
9. Carefully remove the ramekins from the pot. Cool, covered, for 5 minutes.
10. Run a small silicone spatula or a knife around the edge of each ramekin. Invert each quiche onto a small plate and serve.

Substitution tip: Crab also works well in these quiche cups as a substitute for the smoked salmon. Use a seafood seasoning such as Old Bay® instead of the dill.

PREP TIME:
15 minutes

COOK SETTING:
High

PRESSURE-UP TIME: 5 minutes

COOK TIME:
15 minutes

RELEASE: Quick

TOTAL TIME:
41 minutes

SPECIAL EQUIPMENT:
2 (4-inch, 7-ounce) heatproof ramekins

20-MINUTES-OR-LESS PREP

GLUTEN FREE

LOW CARB

PER SERVING:
Calories: 180;
Total Fat: 9g; Protein: 20g;
Carbohydrates: 3g;
Sugars: 1g; Fiber: 1g;
Sodium: 646mg

Shakshuka with Swiss Chard

SERVES 4 (11G CARBS PER SERVING)

PREP TIME:
15 minutes

COOK SETTINGS:
Sauté, Low

SAUTÉ TIME:
10 minutes

PRESSURE-UP TIME: 10 minutes

COOK TIME:
0 minutes

RELEASE: Quick

TOTAL TIME:
37 minutes

SPECIAL EQUIPMENT:
custard cup or
small bowl

20-MINUTES-OR-LESS PREP

GLUTEN FREE

FAMILY FRIENDLY

PER SERVING:
Calories: 182;
Total Fat: 12g; Protein: 8g;
Carbohydrates: 11g;
Sugars: 6g; Fiber: 3g;
Sodium: 851mg

Need a great brunch option? Try shakshuka, a dish where eggs are cooked in seasoned tomato sauce. This version leans toward the Mediterranean with flavors of basil, oregano, garlic, thyme, rosemary, and marjoram. Your EPC needs to be at low pressure for this recipe; the first time I made it, I used high pressure and my eggs ended up overcooked. Look for a pasta sauce that's low in sugar and sodium (or make your own).

4 ounces Swiss chard (about 4 large stems and leaves)

2 tablespoons extra-virgin olive oil

½ medium onion, chopped

½ teaspoon kosher salt

½ teaspoon freshly ground black pepper

½ tablespoon Italian seasoning

2 teaspoons minced garlic

1½ cups Marinara Sauce with Red Lentils (page 124) or tomato-based pasta sauce

4 large eggs

1 tablespoon chopped fresh parsley

2 tablespoons freshly grated Parmesan cheese

1. Separate the stems from the leaves of the Swiss chard. Finely chop the stems; you'll need about ½ cup. Stack the leaves, slice into thin strips, then chop. Set aside.

2. Set the electric pressure cooker to the Sauté setting. When the pot is hot, pour in the olive oil.

3. Add the Swiss chard stems, onion, salt, pepper, and Italian seasoning to the pot, and sauté for 3 to 5 minutes or until the vegetables begin to soften.

4. Add the Swiss chard leaves and garlic, and sauté for 2 more minutes.

5. Hit Cancel. Add the pasta sauce and let the pot cool for 5 minutes.

6. Make 4 evenly spaced indentions in the sauce mixture. Carefully crack an egg into a custard cup, then pour it into one of the indentions. Repeat with the remaining eggs. (Note you can crack the eggs directly into the pot, but the whites will spread out more and the eggs won't look as nice.)

7. Close and lock the lid of the pressure cooker. Set the valve to sealing.

8. Select low pressure and set the timer for 0 minutes.

9. When the cooking is complete, hit Cancel and quick release the pressure.

10. Once the pin drops, unlock and remove the lid.

11. Sprinkle with parsley and Parmesan, and serve immediately.

Substitution tip: If you don't have any Swiss chard, use ½ cup of chopped bell pepper to replace the stems and 2 cups of kale or spinach to replace the leaves.

Hard-boiled Eggs

SERVES 9 (1G CARBS PER SERVING)

Hard-boiling eggs in an EPC removes the guesswork. The eggs come out perfectly cooked and are extremely easy to peel without needing time in an ice water bath after cooking. I like to stand the eggs, larger ends down, in a silicone egg rack that has nine slots. This helps keep the yolks centered. This recipe can be used for as few as three eggs and as many as a dozen.

9 large eggs

1. Pour 1 cup of water into the electric pressure cooker and insert an egg rack. Gently stand the eggs in the rack, fat ends down. If you don't have an egg rack, place the eggs in a steamer basket or on a wire rack.
2. Close and lock the lid of the pressure cooker. Set the valve to sealing.
3. Cook on high pressure for 2 minutes.
4. When the cooking is complete, hit Cancel and allow the pressure to release naturally.
5. Once the pin drops, unlock and remove the lid.
6. Using tongs, carefully remove the eggs from the pressure cooker. Peel or refrigerate the eggs when they are cool enough to handle.

Repurpose tip: Cook a few extra eggs so you can make Guacamole Deviled Eggs: Slice the eggs in half lengthwise, remove the yolks, mash them, and mix with a little guacamole. Stuff the cooked egg whites with the guacamole mixture, sprinkle with chili powder, and enjoy.

PREP TIME:
2 minutes

COOK SETTING:
High

PRESSURE-UP TIME: 6 minutes

COOK TIME:
2 minutes

RELEASE: Natural

RELEASE TIME:
5 minutes

TOTAL TIME:
15 minutes

SPECIAL EQUIPMENT:
egg rack

20-MINUTES-OR-LESS PREP

GLUTEN FREE

LOW CARB

FAMILY FRIENDLY

LOW SODIUM

PER SERVING:
Calories: 78;
Total Fat: 5g; Protein: 6g;
Carbohydrates: 1g;
Sugars: 0.6g; Fiber: 0g;
Sodium: 62mg

PREP TIME:
5 minutes

COOK SETTING:
High

**PRESSURE-UP
TIME:** 5 minutes

COOK TIME:
5 minutes

RELEASE: Quick

TOTAL TIME:
16 minutes

**SPECIAL
EQUIPMENT:**
1 (7-count) silicone
egg bite mold

20-MINUTES-OR-
LESS PREP

GLUTEN FREE

LOW CARB

FAMILY FRIENDLY

LOW SODIUM

PER SERVING:
Calories: 78;
Total Fat: 5g; Protein: 6g;
Carbohydrates: 1g;
Sugars: 0.6g; Fiber: 0g;
Sodium: 62mg

Poached Eggs

SERVES 4 (1G CARBS PER SERVING)

Poaching an egg can be tricky, and all the foodie experts have different advice. Alton Brown says to add vinegar and get your water spinning around before you add the egg. Michael Ruhlman says you need a special perforated spoon to get rid of the "flyaway" whites. Avoid the fuss and "poach" eggs in your pressure cooker instead. It's fast and virtually foolproof. If you like your yolks less runny, cook your eggs an additional minute. This recipe should work for two to seven eggs.

Nonstick cooking spray   4 large eggs

1. Lightly spray 4 cups of a 7-count silicone egg bite mold with nonstick cooking spray. Crack each egg into a sprayed cup.
2. Pour 1 cup of water into the electric pressure cooker. Place the egg bite mold on the wire rack and carefully lower it into the pot.
3. Close and lock the lid of the pressure cooker. Set the valve to sealing.
4. Cook on high pressure for 5 minutes.
5. When the cooking is complete, hit Cancel and quick release the pressure.
6. Once the pin drops, unlock and remove the lid.
7. Run a small rubber spatula or spoon around each egg and carefully remove it from the mold. The white should be cooked, but the yolk should be runny.
8. Serve immediately.

Repurpose tip: Poached eggs are most often eaten atop English muffins with Canadian bacon and hollandaise sauce as "eggs Benedict." However, you can serve them in more creative ways. Top a black bean burger with a poached egg and drizzle with Sriracha sauce. Try one on a piece of avocado toast (using whole grain bread, of course). One of my husband's favorite breakfasts is Lentils with Carrots (page 61) topped with a poached egg. Use your imagination.

Tropical Steel Cut Oats

SERVES 4 (14G CARBS PER SERVING)

Steel cut oats are digested more slowly than other varieties, which is better for your blood sugar. Pressure cooking steel cut oats makes them creamy but allows them to retain their great chewy texture. Try Moxy Kitchen's Spicy Cinnamon Mix as a topping; it's a combination of cinnamon, nutmeg, chili powder, allspice, and ginger. (Moxy makes spice blends that have no added sugar or salt. Their proceeds benefit diabetes research, by the way.)

1 cup steel cut oats

1 cup unsweetened almond milk

2 cups coconut water or water

¾ cup frozen chopped peaches

¾ cup frozen mango chunks

1 (2-inch) vanilla bean, scraped (seeds and pod)

Ground cinnamon

¼ cup chopped unsalted macadamia nuts

1. In the electric pressure cooker, combine the oats, almond milk, coconut water, peaches, mango chunks, and vanilla bean seeds and pod. Stir well.
2. Close and lock the lid of the pressure cooker. Set the valve to sealing.
3. Cook on high pressure for 5 minutes.
4. When the cooking is complete, allow the pressure to release naturally for 10 minutes, then quick release any remaining pressure. Hit Cancel.
5. Once the pin drops, unlock and remove the lid.
6. Discard the vanilla bean pod and stir well.
7. Spoon the oats into 4 bowls. Top each serving with a sprinkle of cinnamon and 1 tablespoon of the macadamia nuts.

Substitution tip: No vanilla bean? Substitute 1 teaspoon of vanilla extract. Peaches in season? Chop two large peaches and use them instead of the frozen peaches and mango chunks. Coconut milk would be a fine replacement for the almond milk but will add more fat. Stay away from cow's milk in this recipe—it will curdle.

PREP TIME:
5 minutes

COOK SETTING:
High

PRESSURE-UP TIME: 14 minutes

COOK TIME:
5 minutes

RELEASE: Natural for 10 minutes, then Quick

TOTAL TIME:
35 minutes

20-MINUTES-OR-LESS PREP

VEGAN

FAMILY FRIENDLY

PER SERVING
(¾ **CUP**): Calories: 127; Total Fat: 7g; Protein: 2g; Carbohydrates: 14g; Sugars: 8g; Fiber: 3g; Sodium: 167mg (with coconut water)

Blueberry Oat Mini Muffins

SERVES 7 (15G CARBS PER SERVING)

PREP TIME:
12 minutes

COOK SETTING:
High

**PRESSURE-UP
TIME:** 8 minutes

COOK TIME:
10 minutes

RELEASE:
Natural for 10 minutes,
then Quick

TOTAL TIME:
46 minutes

**SPECIAL
EQUIPMENT:**
1 (7-count) silicone
egg bite mold

20-MINUTES-OR-
LESS PREP

FAMILY FRIENDLY

LOW SODIUM

PER SERVING:
Calories: 117;
Total Fat: 4g; Protein: 5g;
Carbohydrates: 15g;
Sugars: 4g; Fiber: 2g;
Sodium: 89mg

These muffins don't get brown like baked ones do, but they are still bursting with flavor. Feel free to substitute other berries for the blueberries. You can use fresh instead of frozen berries, but I've found they tend to collect at the bottom of the muffins instead of being evenly distributed throughout. I have heard, but not confirmed, that dark chocolate chips are great instead of berries, too. Add some nuts for crunch, if you'd like.

½ cup rolled oats

¼ cup whole wheat pastry flour or white whole wheat flour

½ tablespoon baking powder

½ teaspoon ground cardamom or ground cinnamon

⅛ teaspoon kosher salt

2 large eggs

½ cup plain Greek yogurt

2 tablespoons pure maple syrup

2 teaspoons extra-virgin olive oil

½ teaspoon vanilla extract

½ cup frozen blueberries (preferably small wild blueberries)

1. In a large bowl, stir together the oats, flour, baking powder, cardamom, and salt.

2. In a medium bowl, whisk together the eggs, yogurt, maple syrup, oil, and vanilla.

3. Add the egg mixture to oat mixture and stir just until combined. Gently fold in the blueberries.

4. Scoop the batter into each cup of the egg bite mold.

5. Pour 1 cup of water into the electric pressure cooker. Place the egg bite mold on the wire rack and carefully lower it into the pot.

6. Close and lock the lid of the pressure cooker. Set the valve to sealing.

7. Cook on high pressure for 10 minutes.

8. When the cooking is complete, allow the pressure to release naturally for 10 minutes, then quick release any remaining pressure. Hit Cancel.

9. Lift the wire rack out of the pot and place on a cooling rack for 5 minutes. Invert the mold onto the cooling rack to release the muffins.

10. Serve the muffins warm or refrigerate or freeze.

Make-ahead tip: Make these muffins ahead of time for a quick, portable snack. You can reheat them in the microwave or simply eat them at room temperature. If you plan to reheat them, hit Cancel before you do the natural release in step 8.

Breakfast Farro with Berries and Walnuts

SERVES 6 (32G CARBS PER SERVING)

While delicious served with berries, this breakfast farro is also quite tasty when topped with almonds and Spiced Pear Applesauce (page 105) or the apples from the Apple Crunch (page 104). If the farro seems too soupy, stir it well and let it sit for a few minutes to absorb more of the liquid.

1 cup farro, rinsed and drained

1 cup unsweetened almond milk

¼ teaspoon kosher salt

½ teaspoon pure vanilla extract

1 teaspoon ground cinnamon

1 tablespoon pure maple syrup

1½ cups fresh blueberries, raspberries, or strawberries (or a combination)

6 tablespoons chopped walnuts

1. In the electric pressure cooker, combine the farro, almond milk, 1 cup of water, salt, vanilla, cinnamon, and maple syrup.
2. Close and lock the lid. Set the valve to sealing.
3. Cook on high pressure for 10 minutes.
4. When the cooking is complete, allow the pressure to release naturally for 10 minutes, then quick release any remaining pressure. Hit Cancel.
5. Once the pin drops, unlock and remove the lid.
6. Stir the farro. Spoon into bowls and top each serving with ¼ cup of berries and 1 tablespoon of walnuts.

Ingredient tip: Farro is a whole wheat grain that's packed with fiber, protein, antioxidants, vitamins, and minerals. "Farro" is an Italian word that can be used to refer to three different types of wheat: emmer, spelt, or einkorn. Most farro sold in the United States is the emmer variety. Cooked farro is similar in texture to barley and has a nutty flavor. Farro is *not* a gluten-free grain.

PREP TIME:
8 minutes

COOK SETTING:
High

PRESSURE-UP TIME: 7 minutes

COOK TIME:
10 minutes

RELEASE: Natural for 10 minutes, then Quick

TOTAL TIME:
36 minutes

20-MINUTES-OR-LESS PREP

VEGAN

FAMILY FRIENDLY

LOW SODIUM

PER SERVING
(⅓ **CUP**): Calories: 189; Total Fat: 5g; Protein: 5g; Carbohydrates: 32g; Sugars: 6g; Fiber: 3g; Sodium: 111mg

PREP TIME:
10 minutes

COOK SETTING:
High

**PRESSURE-UP
TIME:** 7 minutes

COOK TIME:
10 minutes

RELEASE: Quick

TOTAL TIME:
28 minutes

**20-MINUTES-OR-
LESS PREP**

GLUTEN FREE

FAMILY FRIENDLY

LOW SODIUM

PER SERVING
(½ **CUP**): Calories: 218;
Total Fat: 10g; Protein: 5g;
Carbohydrates: 32g;
Sugars: 7g; Fiber: 4g;
Sodium: 28mg

Cranberry Almond Grits

SERVES 5 (32G CARBS PER SERVING)

This recipe turned my Connecticut-born husband into a grits fan. For those of you who think grits are too mushy, you may like this version because the cranberries and toasted almonds add texture. Serve these grits with some protein like Hard-boiled Eggs (page 21) or turkey sausage for breakfast or as a side with pork tenderloin and a green vegetable for dinner.

¾ cup stone-ground grits or polenta (not instant)

½ cup unsweetened dried cranberries

Pinch kosher salt

1 tablespoon unsalted butter or ghee (optional)

1 tablespoon half-and-half

¼ cup sliced almonds, toasted (see page 120)

1. In the electric pressure cooker, stir together the grits, cranberries, salt, and 3 cups of water.

2. Close and lock the lid. Set the valve to sealing.

3. Cook on high pressure for 10 minutes.

4. When the cooking is complete, hit Cancel and quick release the pressure.

5. Once the pin drops, unlock and remove the lid.

6. Add the butter (if using) and half-and-half. Stir until the mixture is creamy, adding more half-and-half if necessary.

7. Spoon into serving bowls and sprinkle with almonds.

Ingredient tip: What's the difference between grits, polenta, and cornmeal? All three are made from ground corn, but grits and polenta tend to be much coarser than cornmeal. Southern-style grits are usually ground from white corn or hominy. Polenta is ground from yellow corn. Good quality stone-ground white grits or yellow polenta can be used in this recipe. (I like the ones from Bob's Red Mill.) "Instant" and "quick-cooking" grits are highly processed and precooked. Do not use them in this recipe.

6-Grain Porridge

SERVES 7 (51G CARBS PER SERVING)

This porridge is an extremely flexible way to add whole grains to your diet. You can use a brown rice/wild rice blend or use a different combination of grains entirely (you'll need about 3 cups total). Top the porridge with any combination of fruit, milk, nuts, and seeds, and add a touch of maple syrup or another sweetener if you'd like. My favorite topping combination is cinnamon, blueberries, raspberries, walnuts, and almond milk.

½ cup steel cut oats

½ cup short-grain brown rice

½ cup millet

½ cup barley

⅓ cup wild rice

¼ cup corn grits or polenta (not instant)

3 tablespoons ground flaxseed

½ teaspoon salt

Ground cinnamon (optional)

Unsweetened almond milk (optional)

Berries (optional)

Sliced almonds or chopped walnuts (optional)

1. In the electric pressure cooker, combine the oats, brown rice, millet, barley, wild rice, grits, flaxseed, salt, and 8 cups of water.
2. Close and lock the lid of the pressure cooker. Set the valve to sealing.
3. Cook on high pressure for 20 minutes.
4. When the cooking is complete, hit Cancel and allow the pressure to release naturally for 15 minutes, then quick release any remaining pressure.
5. Once the pin drops, unlock and remove the lid. Stir.
6. Serve with any combination of cinnamon, almond milk, berries, and nuts (if using).

Leftover tip: This porridge reheats well in the microwave. Make a pot on the weekend and you'll have breakfast in a flash during the busy work week. You can also serve leftovers as a whole grain side dish for dinner.

PREP TIME:
5 minutes

COOK SETTING:
High

PRESSURE-UP TIME: 22 minutes

COOK TIME:
20 minutes

RELEASE: Natural for 15 minutes, then Quick

TOTAL TIME:
1 hour 4 minutes

20-MINUTES-OR-LESS PREP

VEGAN

SUGAR FREE

FAMILY FRIENDLY

LOW SODIUM

PER SERVING
(½ **CUP**): Calories: 263; Total Fat: 3g; Protein: 8g; Carbohydrates: 51g; Sugars: 0.4g; Fiber: 7g; Sodium: 140mg

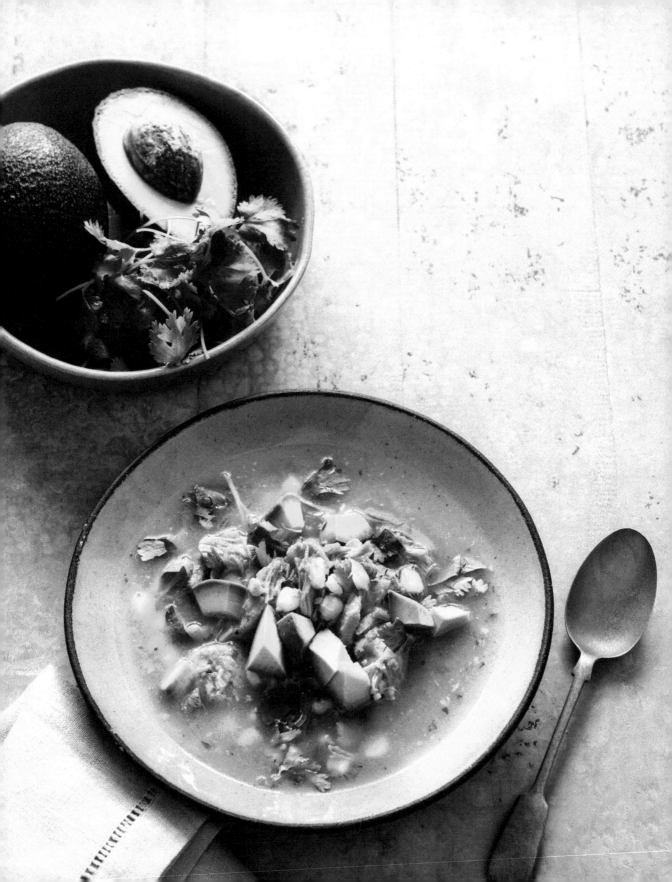

3

Sides and Soups

Parmesan Cauliflower Mash

SERVES 4 (12G CARBS PER SERVING)

PREP TIME:
7 minutes

COOK SETTING:
High

**PRESSURE-UP
TIME:** 18 minutes

COOK TIME:
5 minutes

RELEASE: Quick

TOTAL TIME:
37 minutes

**SPECIAL
EQUIPMENT:**
immersion blender

20-MINUTES-OR-
LESS PREP

GLUTEN FREE

FAMILY FRIENDLY

PER SERVING:
Calories: 141;
Total Fat: 6g; Protein: 12g;
Carbohydrates: 12g;
Sugars: 5g; Fiber: 4g;
Sodium: 592mg

I first discovered cauliflower mash when I tried the South Beach Diet's "surprise" mashed potatoes many years ago. Here, I've swapped the non-butter spray and the fat-free half-and-half for plain Greek yogurt and freshly grated Parmesan cheese. If you prefer a chunky texture, use a potato masher in step 7. If you want a smooth and creamy mash, use an immersion blender or food processor.

1 head cauliflower, cored and cut into large florets

½ teaspoon kosher salt

½ teaspoon garlic pepper

2 tablespoons plain Greek yogurt

¾ cup freshly grated Parmesan cheese

1 tablespoon unsalted butter or ghee (optional)

Chopped fresh chives

1. Pour 1 cup of water into the electric pressure cooker and insert a steamer basket or wire rack.
2. Place the cauliflower in the basket.
3. Close and lock the lid of the pressure cooker. Set the valve to sealing.
4. Cook on high pressure for 5 minutes.
5. When the cooking is complete, hit Cancel and quick release the pressure.
6. Once the pin drops, unlock and remove the lid.
7. Remove the cauliflower from the pot and pour out the water. Return the cauliflower to the pot and add the salt, garlic pepper, yogurt, and cheese. Use an immersion blender or potato masher to purée or mash the cauliflower in the pot.
8. Spoon into a serving bowl, and garnish with butter (if using) and chives.

Substitution tip: Not quite ready to switch from mashed potatoes to mashed cauliflower? Try a blend. Use half a head of cauliflower and 1 pound of chopped potatoes in this recipe, and increase the cook time to 7 minutes. Once you get used to eating that combination, make the move to all cauliflower.

Lemony Brussels Sprouts with Poppy Seeds

SERVES 4 (13G CARBS PER SERVING)

Back in the day when the only cooking shows on TV were found on PBS, I was a huge fan of Nathalie Dupree. Nathalie is a down-to-earth Southern chef who always has interesting ideas. One Saturday morning, she paired Brussels sprouts and poppy seeds. It was such a strange combination, I had to try it. And it worked. I've now adapted her idea for the EPC.

1 pound Brussels sprouts

2 tablespoons avocado oil, divided

1 cup Vegetable Broth (page 116) or Chicken Bone Broth (page 117)

1 tablespoon minced garlic

½ teaspoon kosher salt

Freshly ground black pepper

½ medium lemon

½ tablespoon poppy seeds

PREP TIME:
10 minutes

COOK SETTINGS:
Sauté, High

SAUTÉ TIME:
14 minutes

PRESSURE-UP TIME: 5 minutes

COOK TIME:
2 minutes

RELEASE: Quick

TOTAL TIME:
32 minutes

20-MINUTES-OR-LESS PREP

GLUTEN FREE

VEGAN

FAMILY FRIENDLY

PER SERVING:
Calories: 125;
Total Fat: 8g; Protein: 4g;
Carbohydrates: 13g;
Sugars: 3g; Fiber: 5g;
Sodium: 504mg

1. Trim the Brussels sprouts by cutting off the stem ends and removing any loose outer leaves. Cut each in half lengthwise (through the stem).

2. Set the electric pressure cooker to the Sauté/More setting. When the pot is hot, pour in 1 tablespoon of the avocado oil.

3. Add half of the Brussels sprouts to the pot, cut-side down, and let them brown for 3 to 5 minutes without disturbing. Transfer to a bowl and add the remaining tablespoon of avocado oil and the remaining Brussels sprouts to the pot. Hit Cancel and return all of the Brussels sprouts to the pot.

4. Add the broth, garlic, salt, and a few grinds of pepper. Stir to distribute the seasonings.

5. Close and lock the lid of the pressure cooker. Set the valve to sealing.

6. Cook on high pressure for 2 minutes.

7. While the Brussels sprouts are cooking, zest the lemon, then cut it into quarters.

8. When the cooking is complete, hit Cancel and quick release the pressure.

9. Once the pin drops, unlock and remove the lid.

10. Using a slotted spoon, transfer the Brussels sprouts to a serving bowl. Toss with the lemon zest, a squeeze of lemon juice, and the poppy seeds. Serve immediately.

Ingredient tip: While poppy seeds do come from the pods of opium plants, they are safe to eat and free of narcotic side effects. However, consuming foods containing poppy seeds prior to a drug test for opiates may produce false positive test results.

Sweet and Sour Red Cabbage

SERVES 8 (18G CARBS PER SERVING)

PREP TIME:
10 minutes

COOK SETTING:
High

**PRESSURE-UP
TIME:** 18 minutes

COOK TIME:
10 minutes

RELEASE: Quick

TOTAL TIME:
40 minutes

20-MINUTES-OR-
LESS PREP

GLUTEN FREE

VEGAN

FAMILY FRIENDLY

PER SERVING:
Calories: 73;
Total Fat: 0g; Protein: 2g;
Carbohydrates: 18g;
Sugars: 11g; Fiber: 4g;
Sodium: 160mg

Do you enjoy raw cabbage in dishes like slaw, but never think to cook it? Try this easy cooked cabbage recipe. It's heavy on the "sour" because I'm a huge vinegar fan and like things tart. If you don't, cut back on the amount of apple cider vinegar or add a touch of honey to bump up the sweetness. Serve it with Parmesan Cauliflower Mash (page 30) and grilled pork tenderloin for a hearty meal.

2 cups Spiced Pear Applesauce (page 105) or unsweetened applesauce

1 small onion, chopped

½ cup apple cider vinegar

½ teaspoon kosher salt

1 head red cabbage, cored and thinly sliced

1. In the electric pressure cooker, combine the applesauce, onion, vinegar, salt, and 1 cup of water. Stir in the cabbage.
2. Close and lock the lid of the pressure cooker. Set the valve to sealing.
3. Cook on high pressure for 10 minutes.
4. When the cooking is complete, hit Cancel and quick release the pressure.
5. Once the pin drops, unlock and remove the lid.
6. Spoon into a bowl or platter and serve.

Substitution tip: If you have apples on hand, but no applesauce, you can use them instead. Peel and chop the apples, then add them when you stir in the cabbage.

Coffee-Steamed Carrots

SERVES 4 (12G CARBS PER SERVING)

Recently, I read about a West Coast chef who built his reputation by roasting whole carrots on a bed of coffee beans. At first, I thought I would try using water and whole coffee beans in the bottom of the EPC with sliced carrots in a steamer basket above. Then it hit me that I could just use a cup of brewed coffee and skip the basket entirely.

1 cup brewed coffee

1 teaspoon light brown sugar

½ teaspoon kosher salt

Freshly ground black pepper

1 pound baby carrots

Chopped fresh parsley

1 teaspoon grated lemon zest

1. Pour the coffee into the electric pressure cooker. Stir in the brown sugar, salt, and pepper. Add the carrots.
2. Close and lock the lid of the pressure cooker. Set the valve to sealing.
3. Cook on high pressure for 3 minutes.
4. When the cooking is complete, hit Cancel and quick release the pressure.
5. Once the pin drops, unlock and remove the lid.
6. Using a slotted spoon, transfer the carrots to a serving bowl. Sprinkle with the parsley and lemon zest, and serve.

Substitution tip: If you don't have any baby carrots, you can use whole fresh or frozen chopped carrots instead. For fresh carrots, peel and thickly slice them. Experiment with flavored coffee too; hazelnut would be delicious.

PREP TIME:
5 minutes

COOK SETTING:
High

PRESSURE-UP TIME: 8 minutes

COOK TIME:
3 minutes

RELEASE: Quick

TOTAL TIME:
17 minutes

20-MINUTES-OR-LESS PREP

GLUTEN FREE

VEGAN

PER SERVING:
Calories: 51;
Total Fat: 0g; Protein: 1g;
Carbohydrates: 12g;
Sugars: 7g; Fiber: 4g;
Sodium: 344mg

PREP TIME:
10 minutes

COOK SETTING:
High

**PRESSURE-UP
TIME:** 15 minutes

COOK TIME:
5 minutes

RELEASE: Quick

TOTAL TIME:
30 minutes

20-MINUTES-OR-
LESS PREP

GLUTEN FREE

VEGAN

FAMILY FRIENDLY

LOW SODIUM

**PER SERVING
(½ EAR OF CORN):**
Calories: 62;
Total Fat: 1g; Protein: 2g;
Carbohydrates: 14g;
Sugars: 5g; Fiber: 1g;
Sodium: 11mg

Corn on the Cob

SERVES 12 (14G CARBS PER SERVING)

Do you have the impression that corn is off-limits for people with diabetes? I usually avoid it, but in the summer when the "corn man" at the farmers' market says his corn was just picked that morning, I can't resist. Half an ear (the serving size here) has about 15 grams of carbs, which I can manage. Cooking corn on the cob in an EPC is much easier than boiling or grilling, especially when you're feeding a crowd.

6 ears corn

1. Remove the husks and silk from the corn. Cut or break each ear in half.
2. Pour 1 cup of water into the bottom of the electric pressure cooker. Insert a wire rack or trivet.
3. Place the corn upright on the rack, cut-side down. Close and lock the lid of the pressure cooker. Set the valve to sealing.
4. Cook on high pressure for 5 minutes.
5. When the cooking is complete, hit Cancel and quick release the pressure.
6. Once the pin drops, unlock and remove the lid.
7. Use tongs to remove the corn from the pot. Season as desired and serve immediately.

Leftover tip: Leftover corn? Cut it off the cob and add cooked black beans, diced red bell pepper, avocado chunks, and your favorite vinaigrette for a tasty, high-fiber, meatless lunch.

Parmesan-Topped Acorn Squash

SERVES 4 (12G CARBS PER SERVING)

Acorn squash is a winter squash that's shaped like, well, an acorn. Most have dark green skin, but you may get lucky and snag one that's pale yellow or vibrant orange. Those have thinner skin and moister flesh. Acorn squash is often served with something sweet, like brown sugar or maple syrup. You can avoid those extra carbs by topping off your squash with nutty Parmesan cheese instead. No sweetener required.

1 acorn squash (about 1 pound)

1 tablespoon extra-virgin olive oil

1 teaspoon dried sage leaves, crumbled

¼ teaspoon freshly grated nutmeg

⅛ teaspoon kosher salt

⅛ teaspoon freshly ground black pepper

2 tablespoons freshly grated Parmesan cheese

1. Cut the acorn squash in half lengthwise and remove the seeds. Cut each half in half for a total of 4 wedges. Snap off the stem if it's easy to do.

2. In a small bowl, combine the olive oil, sage, nutmeg, salt, and pepper. Brush the cut sides of the squash with the olive oil mixture.

3. Pour 1 cup of water into the electric pressure cooker and insert a wire rack or trivet.

4. Place the squash on the trivet in a single layer, skin-side down.

5. Close and lock the lid of the pressure cooker. Set the valve to sealing.

6. Cook on high pressure for 20 minutes.

7. When the cooking is complete, hit Cancel and quick release the pressure.

8. Once the pin drops, unlock and remove the lid.

9. Carefully remove the squash from the pot, sprinkle with the Parmesan, and serve.

Substitution tip: If you don't have any whole nutmeg, ground nutmeg will do. You could also try pumpkin pie spice or cinnamon.

PREP TIME:
10 minutes

COOK SETTING:
High

PRESSURE-UP TIME: 10 minutes

COOK TIME:
20 minutes

RELEASE: Quick

TOTAL TIME:
41 minutes

SPECIAL EQUIPMENT:
Microplane grater

20-MINUTES-OR-LESS PREP

GLUTEN FREE

SUGAR FREE

FAMILY FRIENDLY

PER SERVING:
Calories: 85;
Total Fat: 4g; Protein: 2g;
Carbohydrates: 12g;
Sugars: 0g; Fiber: 2g;
Sodium: 282mg

Spaghetti Squash

SERVES 4 (3G CARBS PER SERVING)

Spaghetti squash, a low-carb substitute for pasta, is easy to cook in an EPC. The only tricky part is making sure your squash is small enough to fit inside the pot. Cutting the squash crosswise instead of lengthwise results in longer strands of "spaghetti." Simply top the squash with a little salt, garlic pepper, and Parmesan for a quick side.

1 spaghetti squash (about 2 pounds)

1. Cut the spaghetti squash in half crosswise and use a large spoon to remove the seeds.
2. Pour 1 cup of water into the electric pressure cooker and insert a wire rack or trivet.
3. Place the squash halves on the rack, cut-side up.
4. Close and lock the lid of the pressure cooker. Set the valve to sealing.
5. Cook on high pressure for 7 minutes.
6. When the cooking is complete, hit Cancel and quick release the pressure.
7. Once the pin drops, unlock and remove the lid.
8. With tongs, remove the squash from the pot and transfer it to a plate. When it is cool enough to handle, scrape the squash with the tines of a fork to remove the strands. Discard the skin.

Make-ahead tip: Prepare the spaghetti squash and refrigerate the strands. Reheat it in the microwave and serve alongside Marinara Sauce with Red Lentils (page 124), or as a substitute for pasta in your favorite pasta dish. Other ways to eat spaghetti squash include: a substitute for noodles in a casserole; a bed for sautéed vegetables; or topped with fresh diced tomatoes, feta cheese, and basil.

PREP TIME:
5 minutes

COOK SETTING:
High

PRESSURE-UP TIME: 12 minutes

COOK TIME:
7 minutes

RELEASE: Quick

TOTAL TIME:
30 minutes

20-MINUTES-OR-LESS PREP

GLUTEN FREE

VEGAN

LOW CARB

FAMILY FRIENDLY

LOW SODIUM

PER SERVING:
Calories: 10;
Total Fat: 0g; Protein: 0g;
Carbohydrates: 3g;
Sugars: 1g; Fiber: 1g;
Sodium: 17mg

Buttercup Squash Soup

SERVES 6 (18G CARBS PER SERVING)

I like this soup served hot, but I love it when it's cold. In fact, I've been known to drink it at breakfast to sneak in some veggies or slurp some down as a quick snack before heading to the gym. Freshly grated nutmeg is perfect here, but remember, a little goes a long way. Use white pepper instead of black so your soup doesn't have dark specks in it.

2 tablespoons extra-virgin olive oil

1 medium onion, chopped

4 to 5 cups Vegetable Broth (page 116) or Chicken Bone Broth (page 117)

1½ pounds buttercup squash, peeled, seeded, and cut into 1-inch chunks

½ teaspoon kosher salt

¼ teaspoon ground white pepper

Whole nutmeg, for grating

1. Set the electric pressure cooker to the Sauté setting. When the pot is hot, pour in the olive oil.

2. Add the onion and sauté for 3 to 5 minutes, until it begins to soften. Hit Cancel.

3. Add the broth, squash, salt, and pepper to the pot and stir. (If you want a thicker soup, use 4 cups of broth. If you want a thinner, drinkable soup, use 5 cups.)

4. Close and lock the lid of the pressure cooker. Set the valve to sealing.

5. Cook on high pressure for 10 minutes.

6. When the cooking is complete, hit Cancel and allow the pressure to release naturally.

7. Once the pin drops, unlock and remove the lid.

8. Use an immersion blender to purée the soup right in the pot. If you don't have an immersion blender, transfer the soup to a blender or food processor and purée. (Follow the instructions that came with your machine for blending hot foods.)

9. Pour the soup into serving bowls and grate nutmeg on top.

Substitution tip: Buttercup squash looks like a speckled, compressed, green pumpkin and is a bit sweeter than most winter squash. If you can't find it, butternut will work just fine. You can often find precut fresh or frozen butternut squash, which will save you some prep time.

PREP TIME:
15 minutes

COOK SETTINGS:
Sauté, High

SAUTÉ TIME:
5 minutes

PRESSURE-UP TIME: 15 minutes

COOK TIME:
10 minutes

RELEASE: Natural

TOTAL TIME:
1 hour 4 minutes

SPECIAL EQUIPMENT:
immersion blender, blender, or food processor; Microplane grater

20-MINUTES-OR-LESS PREP

GLUTEN FREE

VEGAN

FAMILY FRIENDLY

PER SERVING (1⅓ CUPS):
Calories: 110;
Total Fat: 5g; Protein: 1g;
Carbohydrates: 18g;
Sugars: 4g; Fiber: 4g;
Sodium: 166mg

PREP TIME:
10 minutes

COOK SETTING:
High

**PRESSURE-UP
TIME:** 11 minutes

COOK TIME:
25 minutes

RELEASE: Natural
for 15 minutes,
then Quick

TOTAL TIME:
1 hour 7 minutes

**SPECIAL
EQUIPMENT:**
small jar with
screw-top lid

20-MINUTES-OR-
LESS PREP

GLUTEN FREE

FAMILY FRIENDLY

LOW SODIUM

PER SERVING
(⅓ **CUP**): Calories: 126;
Total Fat: 5g; Protein: 3g;
Carbohydrates: 18g;
Sugars: 2g; Fiber: 2g;
Sodium: 120mg

Wild Rice Salad with Cranberries and Almonds

SERVES 18 (18G CARBS PER SERVING)

Any wild rice blend should work in this recipe; I like Lundberg's Wild Blend Rice, which includes a combination of brown, wild, and black rice. (Avoid white rice if you can.) This salad, a great potluck dish, is very versatile. Feel free to use another type of dried fruit or nut and serve it warm, cold, or at room temperature. You can make this salad vegan if you use vegetable broth and maple syrup.

For the rice

2 cups wild rice blend, rinsed

1 teaspoon kosher salt

2½ cups Vegetable Broth (page 116) or Chicken Bone Broth (page 117)

For the dressing

¼ cup extra-virgin olive oil

¼ cup white wine vinegar

1½ teaspoons grated orange zest

Juice of 1 medium orange (about ¼ cup)

1 teaspoon honey or pure maple syrup

For the salad

¾ cup unsweetened dried cranberries

½ cup sliced almonds, toasted (see page 120)

Freshly ground black pepper

To make the rice

1. In the electric pressure cooker, combine the rice, salt, and broth.

2. Close and lock the lid. Set the valve to sealing.

3. Cook on high pressure for 25 minutes.

4. When the cooking is complete, hit Cancel and allow the pressure to release naturally for 15 minutes, then quick release any remaining pressure.

5. Once the pin drops, unlock and remove the lid.

6. Let the rice cool briefly, then fluff it with a fork.

To make the dressing

While the rice cooks, make the dressing: In a small jar with a screw-top lid, combine the olive oil, vinegar, zest, juice, and honey. (If you don't have a jar, whisk the ingredients together in a small bowl.) Shake to combine.

To make the salad

1. In a large bowl, combine the rice, cranberries, and almonds.
2. Add the dressing and season with pepper.
3. Serve warm or refrigerate.

Make-ahead tip: Cook the wild rice ahead of time and refrigerate. When you're ready to serve the salad, make the dressing, add the cranberries and almonds, and season with pepper. You can also make the whole salad ahead and refrigerate until serving time.

Creamy Sweet Potato Soup

SERVES 6 (36G CARBS PER SERVING)

When you blend this soup, you'll be amazed that it can be so creamy without containing any dairy products. My husband, who often asserts that sweet potatoes are too "earthy," loves this soup. The flavors will remind you of a Thanksgiving sweet potato casserole, minus the marshmallows.

PREP TIME:
15 minutes

COOK SETTINGS:
Sauté, High

SAUTÉ TIME:
9 minutes

PRESSURE-UP TIME: 14 minutes

COOK TIME:
10 minutes

RELEASE: Natural

TOTAL TIME:
1 hour 3 minutes

SPECIAL EQUIPMENT:
immersion blender, blender, or food processor

20-MINUTES-OR-LESS PREP

GLUTEN FREE

VEGAN

FAMILY FRIENDLY

**PER SERVING
(1 CUP):** Calories: 193;
Total Fat: 5g; Protein: 3g;
Carbohydrates: 36g;
Sugars: 8g; Fiber: 6g;
Sodium: 302mg

2 tablespoons avocado oil

1 small onion, chopped

2 celery stalks, chopped

2 teaspoons minced garlic

1 teaspoon kosher salt

½ teaspoon freshly ground black pepper

1 teaspoon ground turmeric

½ teaspoon ground cinnamon

2 pounds sweet potatoes, peeled and cut into 1-inch cubes

3 cups Vegetable Broth (page 116) or Chicken Bone Broth (page 117)

Plain Greek yogurt, to garnish (optional)

Chopped fresh parsley, to garnish (optional)

Pumpkin seeds (pepitas), to garnish (optional)

1. Set the electric pressure cooker to the Sauté setting. When the pot is hot, pour in the avocado oil.

2. Sauté the onion and celery for 3 to 5 minutes or until the vegetables begin to soften.

3. Stir in the garlic, salt, pepper, turmeric, and cinnamon. Hit Cancel.

4. Stir in the sweet potatoes and broth.

5. Close and lock the lid of the pressure cooker. Set the valve to sealing.

6. Cook on high pressure for 10 minutes.

7. When the cooking is complete, hit Cancel and allow the pressure to release naturally.

8. Once the pin drops, unlock and remove the lid.

9. Use an immersion blender to purée the soup right in the pot. If you don't have an immersion blender, transfer the soup to a blender or food processor and purée. (Follow the instructions that came with your machine for blending hot foods.)

10. Spoon into bowls and serve topped with Greek yogurt, parsley, and/or pumpkin seeds (if using).

Ingredient tip: Turmeric, a spice in the ginger family, is a major source of curcumin, a substance that contains antioxidants and is known to have anti-inflammatory properties that benefit conditions such as metabolic syndrome, high cholesterol, and arthritis. To maximize the health benefits of turmeric, eat some black pepper at the same time.

Black Bean Soup with Lime-Yogurt Drizzle

SERVES 8 (42G CARBS PER SERVING)

In this soup, you just throw dried black beans into the pot and they cook perfectly, no soaking required. If you avoid dairy, top the soup with some chopped avocado and a squeeze of lime juice. Even if you do eat dairy, the avocado would be a nice touch. Don't worry about the green chilies; they are very mild. If you want more heat, stir some hot sauce into the lime-yogurt mixture.

2 tablespoons avocado oil

1 medium onion, chopped

3 garlic cloves, minced

1 teaspoon ground cumin

1 (10-ounce) can diced tomatoes and green chilies

6 cups Chicken Bone Broth (page 117), Vegetable Broth (page 116), or water

1 pound dried black beans, rinsed

Kosher salt

¼ cup plain Greek yogurt or sour cream

1 tablespoon freshly squeezed lime juice

1. Set the electric pressure cooker to the Sauté setting. When the pot is hot, pour in the avocado oil.

2. Sauté the onion for 3 to 5 minutes, until it begins to soften. Hit Cancel.

3. Stir in the garlic, cumin, tomatoes and their juices, broth, and beans.

4. Close and lock the lid of the pressure cooker. Set the valve to sealing.

5. Cook on high pressure for 40 minutes.

6. While the soup is cooking, combine the yogurt and lime juice in a small bowl.

7. When the cooking is complete, hit Cancel. Allow the pressure to release naturally for 15 minutes, then quick release any remaining pressure.

8. Once the pin drops, unlock and remove the lid.

9. (Optional) For a thicker soup, remove 1½ cups of beans from the pot using a slotted spoon. Use an immersion blender to blend the beans that remain in the pot. If you don't have an immersion blender, transfer the soup left in the pot to a blender or food processor and purée. (Follow the instructions that came with your machine for blending hot foods.) Stir in the reserved beans. Season with salt, if desired.

10. Spoon into serving bowls and drizzle with lime-yogurt sauce.

Leftover tip: This black bean soup keeps in the refrigerator for about a week and reheats easily, so it's perfect for a quick lunch. It freezes well, too. Don't add the lime-yogurt sauce until you're ready to eat.

PREP TIME:
10 minutes

COOK SETTINGS:
Sauté, High

SAUTÉ TIME:
5 minutes

PRESSURE-UP TIME: 17 minutes

COOK TIME:
40 minutes

RELEASE: Natural for 15 minutes, then Quick

TOTAL TIME:
1 hour 28 minutes

SPECIAL EQUIPMENT:
immersion blender, blender, or food processor

20-MINUTES-OR-LESS PREP

GLUTEN FREE

FAMILY FRIENDLY

PER SERVING (1 CUP): Calories: 285; Total Fat: 6g; Protein: 19g; Carbohydrates: 42g; Sugars: 3g; Fiber: 10g; Sodium: 174mg

Chicken Noodle Soup

SERVES 12 (17G CARBS PER SERVING)

PREP TIME:
15 minutes

COOK SETTINGS:
Sauté, High

SAUTÉ TIME:
5 minutes + 5 minutes

**PRESSURE-UP
TIME:** 31 minutes

COOK TIME:
20 minutes

RELEASE: Quick

TOTAL TIME:
1 hour 32 minutes

20-MINUTES-OR-
LESS PREP

FAMILY FRIENDLY

**PER SERVING
(1 CUP):** Calories: 330;
Total Fat: 15g; Protein: 32g;
Carbohydrates: 17g;
Sugars: 3g; Fiber: 4g;
Sodium: 451mg

Sometimes you just need a bowl of chicken noodle soup, and in an EPC, it's easy. Homemade soup also allows you to control the chicken-to-noodle balance for a lower-carb option. My mom, who was on a soft foods diet after some dental surgery, confirms that this soup is delicious even after being puréed in a blender.

2 tablespoons avocado oil

1 medium onion, chopped

3 celery stalks, chopped

1 teaspoon kosher salt

¼ teaspoon freshly ground
   black pepper

2 teaspoons minced garlic

5 large carrots, peeled and cut into
   ¼-inch-thick rounds

3 pounds bone-in chicken breasts
   (about 3)

4 cups Chicken Bone Broth
   (page 117) or low-sodium
   store-bought chicken broth

4 cups water

2 tablespoons soy sauce

6 ounces whole grain wide
   egg noodles

1. Set the electric pressure cooker to the Sauté setting. When the pot is hot, pour in the avocado oil.

2. Sauté the onion, celery, salt, and pepper for 3 to 5 minutes or until the vegetables begin to soften.

3. Add the garlic and carrots, and stir to mix well. Hit Cancel.

4. Add the chicken to the pot, meat-side down. Add the broth, water, and soy sauce. Close and lock the lid of the pressure cooker. Set the valve to sealing.

5. Cook on high pressure for 20 minutes.

6. When the cooking is complete, hit Cancel and quick release the pressure. Unlock and remove the lid.

7. Using tongs, remove the chicken breasts to a cutting board. Hit Sauté/More and bring the soup to a boil.

8. Add the noodles and cook for 4 to 5 minutes or until the noodles are al dente.

9. While the noodles are cooking, use two forks to shred the chicken. Add the meat back to the pot and save the bones to make more bone broth.

10. Season with additional pepper, if desired, and serve.

Leftover tip: If you want to freeze the soup, don't add the noodles before freezing. Prepare the recipe through step 6, remove the chicken and shred it, then add the chicken back into the soup. Cool and freeze. When ready to eat, thaw the soup, bring it to a boil, and add the noodles. Cook until the noodles are al dente, and serve. You could also skip the noodles entirely or add in leftover rice or pasta.

Turkey Barley Vegetable Soup

SERVES 8 (21G CARBS PER SERVING)

PREP TIME:
5 minutes

COOK SETTINGS:
Sauté, High

SAUTÉ TIME:
10 minutes

**PRESSURE-UP
TIME:** 25 minutes

COOK TIME:
20 minutes

RELEASE: Natural
for 10 minutes,
then Quick

TOTAL TIME:
1 hour 12 minutes

20-MINUTES-OR-
LESS PREP

FAMILY FRIENDLY

PER SERVING
(1¼ **CUP):** Calories: 253;
Total Fat: 12g; Protein: 19g;
Carbohydrates: 21g;
Sugars: 7g; Fiber: 7g;
Sodium: 560mg

I've been making this soup in various forms since my best friend gave me the recipe more than 30 years ago. The original version contained ground beef, bouillon, and ketchup and was cooked on the stovetop. This revamped version uses lower-fat ground turkey, homemade bone broth, and frozen vegetables, which are convenient and work so well in the EPC.

2 tablespoons avocado oil

1 pound ground turkey

4 cups Chicken Bone Broth (page 117), low-sodium store-bought chicken broth, or water

1 (28-ounce) carton or can diced tomatoes

2 tablespoons tomato paste

1 (15-ounce) package frozen chopped carrots (about 2½ cups)

1 (15-ounce) package frozen peppers and onions (about 2½ cups)

⅓ cup dry barley

1 teaspoon kosher salt

¼ teaspoon freshly ground black pepper

2 bay leaves

1. Set the electric pressure cooker to the Sauté/More setting. When the pot is hot, pour in the avocado oil.
2. Add the turkey to the pot and sauté, stirring frequently to break up the meat, for about 7 minutes or until the turkey is no longer pink. Hit Cancel.
3. Add the broth, tomatoes and their juices, and tomato paste. Stir in the carrots, peppers and onions, barley, salt, pepper, and bay leaves.
4. Close and lock the lid of the pressure cooker. Set the valve to sealing.
5. Cook on high pressure for 20 minutes.
6. When the cooking is complete, hit Cancel and allow the pressure to release naturally for 10 minutes, then quick release any remaining pressure.
7. Once the pin drops, unlock and remove the lid. Discard the bay leaves.
8. Spoon into bowls and serve.

Substitution tip: Ground chicken works fine instead of ground turkey. You can also use fresh sliced carrots and/or chopped peppers and onions. If you use fresh peppers and onions, sauté them along with the turkey.

4-Ingredient Carnitas Posole

SERVES 4 (20G CARBS PER SERVING)

I came up with the idea for this spicy soup when I had some leftover Pork Carnitas (page 94) staring at me every time I opened the refrigerator. If you don't, use any shredded cooked pork or pick up some carnitas at your favorite Mexican restaurant (hold the rice and beans). Not a fan of spicy food? Look for a mild salsa verde or make your own Roasted Tomatillo Salsa (page 121) so you can control the heat.

2 cups Chicken Bone Broth (page 117) or low-sodium store-bought chicken broth

1 (15-ounce) can hominy

2 cups Pork Carnitas (page 94) or shredded cooked pork

2 cups Roasted Tomatillo Salsa (page 121)

Chopped avocado, for serving (optional)

Chopped cilantro, for garnish (optional)

PREP TIME:
5 minutes

COOK SETTING:
High

PRESSURE-UP TIME: 16 minutes

COOK TIME:
8 minutes

RELEASE: Quick

TOTAL TIME:
32 minutes

20-MINUTES-OR-LESS PREP

GLUTEN FREE

FAMILY FRIENDLY

PER SERVING:
Calories: 264;
Total Fat: 7g; Protein: 28g;
Carbohydrates: 20g;
Sugars: 5g; Fiber: 7g;
Sodium: 590mg

1. In the electric pressure cooker, combine the broth, hominy and its juices, pork, and salsa. Stir to combine.
2. Close and lock the lid of the pressure cooker. Set the valve to sealing.
3. Cook on high pressure for 8 minutes.
4. When the cooking is complete, hit Cancel and quick release the pressure.
5. Once the pin drops, unlock and remove the lid.
6. Spoon into bowls and serve with avocado and/or cilantro (if using).

Ingredient tip: Hominy is corn kernels that have been soaked in lye or lime (the mineral) to remove the hulls and germ. It can then be ground to make grits, or cooked until soft and used to thicken soups. Sometimes you can find hominy dried, but mostly you'll see it canned. Dried hominy can be cooked the way you would cook dried beans; canned hominy is already cooked. *Posole* (or *pozole*) is a traditional Mexican soup made with pork and hominy.

Easy tip: If you're pressed for time, you can use a jar (16 ounce) of store-bought salsa verde.

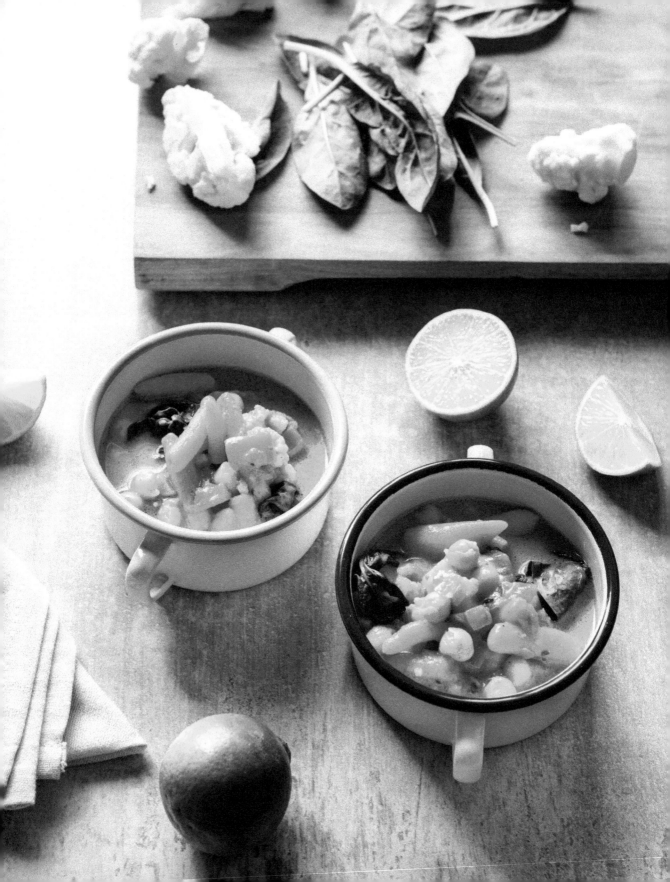

4

Meatless Mains

Strawberry Farro Salad

SERVES 8 (22G CARBS PER SERVING)

PREP TIME:
17 minutes

COOK SETTING:
High

**PRESSURE-UP
TIME:** 8 minutes

COOK TIME:
10 minutes

RELEASE: Natural
for 10 minutes,
then Quick

TOTAL TIME:
50 minutes

**SPECIAL
EQUIPMENT:**
small jar with
screw-top lid

20-MINUTES-OR-
LESS PREP

FAMILY FRIENDLY

LOW SODIUM

PER SERVING
(½ **CUP):** Calories: 176;
Total Fat: 9g; Protein: 3g;
Carbohydrates: 22g;
Sugars: 3g; Fiber: 2g;
Sodium: 68mg

Farro is a high-fiber ancient grain with a surprising amount of protein. This salad is great as a main dish or a side, and I have been known to eat it cold for breakfast, too. It has the best flavor during the summer months when strawberries and basil are both in season. If there appears to be a lot of liquid when you open the pot, don't worry. The farro will absorb more liquid as it cools. Using maple syrup will make this salad vegan.

For the farro

1 cup farro, rinsed and drained

¼ teaspoon kosher salt

For the dressing

1 tablespoon freshly squeezed lime juice (from ½ medium lime)

½ tablespoon fruit-flavored balsamic vinegar

½ teaspoon Dijon mustard

½ tablespoon honey or pure maple syrup

½ teaspoon poppy seeds

¼ cup extra-virgin olive oil

For the salad

1¼ cups sliced strawberries

¼ cup slivered almonds, toasted

Freshly ground black pepper

Fresh basil leaves, cut into a chiffonade, for garnish

To make the farro

1. In the electric pressure cooker, combine the farro, salt, and 2 cups of water.
2. Close and lock the lid. Set the valve to sealing.
3. Cook on high pressure for 10 minutes.
4. When the cooking is complete, allow the pressure to release naturally for 10 minutes, then quick release the remaining pressure. Hit Cancel.
5. Once the pin drops, unlock and remove the lid.
6. Fluff the farro with a fork and let cool.

To make the dressing

While the farro is cooking, in a small jar with a screw-top lid, combine the lime juice, balsamic vinegar, mustard, honey, poppy seeds, and olive oil. Shake until well combined.

To make the salad

1. In a large bowl, toss the farro with the dressing. Stir in the strawberries and almonds.

2. Season with pepper, garnish with basil, and serve.

Make-ahead tip: Cook the farro ahead of time, and store it in the refrigerator until you're ready to serve the salad.

PREP TIME:
15 minutes

COOK SETTING:
High

**PRESSURE-UP
TIME:** 6 minutes

COOK TIME:
22 minutes

RELEASE: Natural
for 10 minutes,
then Quick

TOTAL TIME:
59 minutes

**SPECIAL
EQUIPMENT:**
small jar with
screw-top lid

20-MINUTES-OR-
LESS PREP

GLUTEN FREE

LOW SODIUM

VEGAN

FAMILY FRIENDLY

PER SERVING
(½ **CUP):** Calories: 170;
Total Fat: 11g; Protein: 5g;
Carbohydrates: 15g;
Sugars: 3g; Fiber: 2g;
Sodium: 10mg

Lemony Black Rice Salad with Edamame

SERVES 8 (15G CARBS PER SERVING)

To use a 1:1 ratio of rice to water in the EPC, make sure your rice is wet to start. The rice will come out dry, yet perfectly cooked. This salad comes together quickly. Just make the dressing, thaw the edamame, slice the scallions, and chop the walnuts while the rice is cooking. A note about lemons: the ugly ones are usually the juiciest.

For the rice

1 cup black rice (forbidden rice),
   rinsed and still wet

For the dressing

3 tablespoons extra-virgin olive oil

2 tablespoons freshly squeezed
   lemon juice

2 tablespoons white wine vinegar or
   rice vinegar

1 tablespoon honey or pure
   maple syrup

1 tablespoon sesame oil

For the salad

1 (8-ounce) bag frozen shelled
   edamame, thawed (about 1½ cups)

2 scallions, both white and green
   parts, thinly sliced

¼ cup chopped walnuts

Kosher salt

Freshly ground black pepper

To make the rice

1. In the electric pressure cooker, combine the rice and 1 cup of water.

2. Close and lock the lid of the pressure cooker. Set the valve to sealing.

3. Cook on high pressure for 22 minutes.

4. When the cooking is complete, hit Cancel and allow the pressure to release naturally for 10 minutes, then quick release any remaining pressure.

5. Once the pin drops, unlock and remove the lid.

6. Fluff the rice with a fork and let it cool.

To make the dressing

While the rice is cooking, make the dressing. In a small jar with a screw-top lid, combine the olive oil, lemon juice, vinegar, honey or maple syrup, and sesame oil. Shake until well combined.

To make the salad

1. Shake up the dressing. In a large bowl, toss the rice and dressing. Stir in the edamame, scallions, and walnuts.
2. Season with salt and pepper.

Ingredient tip: Black (forbidden) rice is high in fiber and protein—plus, it's loaded with antioxidants. It contains more protein than brown rice and double the amount found in white rice. A small study has shown that black rice may also help decrease arterial plaque, which will help keep your heart healthy.

Moroccan Eggplant Stew

SERVES 4 (28G CARBS PER SERVING)

PREP TIME:
20 minutes

COOK SETTINGS:
Sauté, High

SAUTÉ TIME:
5 minutes

**PRESSURE-UP
TIME:** 15 minutes

COOK TIME:
3 minutes

RELEASE: Natural

TOTAL TIME:
58 minutes

**20-MINUTES-OR-
LESS PREP**

GLUTEN FREE

VEGAN

FAMILY FRIENDLY

**PER SERVING
(1½ CUPS):**
Calories: 216;
Total Fat: 8g; Protein: 4g;
Carbohydrates: 28g;
Sugars: 9g; Fiber: 8g;
Sodium: 735mg

The only eggplants I'd ever seen before I started frequenting farmers' markets were those fat, dark purple, seedy ones. I wasn't a fan. Once I discovered the round, orange African and skinny, light-purple Asian varieties, I learned I actually liked eggplant. The first time I made this stew, I used tiny pineapple tomatillos (also found at the farmers' market), which didn't even require chopping.

2 tablespoons avocado oil

1 large onion, minced

2 garlic cloves, minced

1 teaspoon ras el hanout spice blend or curry powder

¼ teaspoon cayenne pepper

1 teaspoon kosher salt

1 cup Vegetable Broth (page 116) or water

1 tablespoon tomato paste

2 cups chopped eggplant

2 medium gold potatoes, peeled and chopped

4 ounces tomatillos, husks removed, chopped

1 (14-ounce) can diced tomatoes

1. Set the electric pressure cooker to the Sauté setting. When the pot is hot, pour in the avocado oil.

2. Sauté the onion for 3 to 5 minutes, until it begins to soften. Add the garlic, ras el hanout, cayenne, and salt. Cook and stir for about 30 seconds. Hit Cancel.

3. Stir in the broth and tomato paste. Add the eggplant, potatoes, tomatillos, and tomatoes with their juices.

4. Close and lock the lid of the pressure cooker. Set the valve to sealing.

5. Cook on high pressure for 3 minutes.

6. When the cooking is complete, hit Cancel and allow the pressure to release naturally.

7. Once the pin drops, unlock and remove the lid.

8. Stir well and spoon into serving bowls.

Ingredient: Ras el hanout is a Moroccan spice blend that may feature cardamom, cumin, cloves, cinnamon, nutmeg, mace, allspice, ginger, pepper, paprika, and turmeric. Different brands contain different blends of spices. Think of it as North Africa's garam masala. If you can't find ras el hanout, use curry powder instead.

Mexican Zucchini Casserole

SERVES 4 (23G CARBS PER SERVING)

If you have a mandoline and aren't terrified of it, use it in this recipe to make quick and uniform work of the zucchini. Your rounds will be thinner than if you use a knife, so you may want to include more zucchini slices in each layer. If you have an ovenproof casserole dish that fits inside your EPC, you can use it instead of a cake pan.

1 (6 to 7-inch) zucchini, trimmed

Nonstick cooking spray

1 (15-ounce) can pinto beans or
  1½ cups Salt-Free No-Soak Beans
  (page 64), rinsed and drained

1⅓ cups salsa

1⅓ cups shredded Mexican
  cheese blend

1. Slice the zucchini into rounds. You'll need at least 16 slices.
2. Spray a 6-inch cake pan with nonstick spray.
3. Put the beans into a medium bowl and mash some of them with a fork.
4. Cover the bottom of the pan with about 4 zucchini slices. Add about ⅓ of the beans, ⅓ cup of salsa, and ⅓ cup of cheese. Press down. Repeat for 2 more layers. Add the remaining zucchini, salsa, and cheese. (There are no beans in the top layer.)
5. Cover the pan loosely with foil.
6. Pour 1 cup of water into the electric pressure cooker.
7. Place the pan on the wire rack and carefully lower it into the pot. Close and lock the lid of the pressure cooker. Set the valve to sealing.
8. Cook on high pressure for 15 minutes.
9. When the cooking is complete, hit Cancel and allow the pressure to release naturally.
10. Once the pin drops, unlock and remove the lid.
11. Carefully remove the pan from the pot, lifting by the handles of the wire rack. Let the casserole sit for 5 minutes before slicing into quarters and serving.

Substitution tip: Use any salsa and cheese combination you like. I especially like pineapple salsa with a Monterey Jack/cheddar blend.

PREP TIME:
15 minutes

COOK SETTING:
High

**PRESSURE-UP
TIME:** 9 minutes

COOK TIME:
15 minutes

RELEASE: Natural

TOTAL TIME:
54 minutes

**SPECIAL
EQUIPMENT:**
6-inch cake pan

20-MINUTES-OR-
LESS PREP

GLUTEN FREE

FAMILY FRIENDLY

PER SERVING:
Calories: 252;
Total Fat: 12g; Protein: 16g;
Carbohydrates: 23g;
Sugars: 4g; Fiber: 7g;
Sodium: 1089mg

PREP TIME:
15 minutes

COOK SETTINGS:
Sauté, High

SAUTÉ TIME:
7 minutes

**PRESSURE-UP
TIME:** 14 minutes

COOK TIME:
5 minutes

RELEASE: Quick

TOTAL TIME:
53 minutes

**20-MINUTES-OR-
LESS PREP**

GLUTEN FREE

FAMILY FRIENDLY

**PER SERVING
(1 CUP):** Calories: 152;
Total Fat: 5g; Protein: 6g;
Carbohydrates: 23g;
Sugars: 8g; Fiber: 7g;
Sodium: 357mg

Minestrone with Red Beans, Zucchini, and Spinach

SERVES 8 (23G CARBS PER SERVING)

Minestrone is a thick Italian soup usually made with vegetables, beans, and pasta. This version is extremely flexible; use whatever beans and veggies you like. Whole wheat orzo thickens the soup and provides more bulk to fill you up—but feel free to leave it out if you can't eat pasta.

For the soup

2 tablespoons avocado oil

1 cup chopped onion

1 celery stalk, chopped

1 teaspoon dried thyme

½ teaspoon dried sage leaves

½ teaspoon freshly ground
black pepper

2 cups Vegetable Broth (page 116)
or water

1 (28-ounce) carton or can chopped
tomatoes

1 (15-ounce can) small red beans,
rinsed and drained

2 carrots, peeled and chopped

2 bay leaves

½ cup whole wheat orzo, uncooked
(optional)

For the finish

1 medium zucchini, quartered
lengthwise, then chopped

2 cups baby spinach

¼ cup freshly grated
Parmesan cheese

Chopped fresh basil (optional)

To make the soup

1. Set the electric pressure cooker to the Sauté setting. When the pot is hot, pour in the avocado oil.

2. Sauté the onion and celery for 3 to 5 minutes, or until the vegetables begin to soften. Stir in the thyme, sage, and pepper. Hit Cancel.

3. Add the broth, tomatoes and their juices, beans, carrots, bay leaves, and orzo (if using).

4. Close and lock the lid of the pressure cooker. Set the valve to sealing.

5. Cook on high pressure for 5 minutes.

6. When the cooking is complete, hit Cancel and quick release the pressure.

7. Once the pin drops, unlock and remove the lid.

To finish the soup

1. Stir in the zucchini and spinach. Replace the lid and let the pot sit for 10 minutes.

2. Spoon into serving bowls and top with the Parmesan cheese and basil (if using).

Make-ahead tip: Make the soup through step 7, omitting the orzo. Cool and then freeze or refrigerate. When you're ready to eat the minestrone, reheat it on the stovetop. When the soup comes to a simmer, add the orzo (if using), zucchini, and spinach. Cook until the orzo is al dente, then serve with the Parmesan and basil (if using).

Savory Bread Pudding with Mushrooms and Kale

SERVES 2 (23G CARBS PER SERVING)

PREP TIME:
20 minutes

COOK SETTINGS:
Sauté, High

SAUTÉ TIME:
8 minutes

PRESSURE-UP TIME: 4 minutes

COOK TIME:
8 minutes

RELEASE: Natural for 10 minutes, then Quick

TOTAL TIME:
55 minutes

SPECIAL EQUIPMENT:
2 (4-inch, 7-ounce) heatproof ramekins

20-MINUTES-OR-LESS PREP

PER SERVING:
Calories: 295;
Total Fat: 17g; Protein: 13g;
Carbohydrates: 23g;
Sugars: 7g; Fiber: 3g;
Sodium: 313mg

My mushroom-loving husband often feels deprived. I don't like mushrooms, so I don't cook with them often. When I saw a savory bread pudding recipe featuring mushrooms in a magazine at the doctor's office, I decided to surprise him. I used creminis, but almost any other variety will work just as well.

1 large egg

½ cup 2% milk

½ teaspoon Dijon mustard

Pinch freshly grated nutmeg

Pinch kosher salt

Pinch freshly ground black pepper

1 slice sourdough bread (about 1 ounce), cut into 1-inch cubes

1 tablespoon avocado oil

¼ cup chopped onion

2 ounces mushrooms, sliced (about 3 creminis)

¼ teaspoon dried thyme

1 cup chopped lacinato kale, stems and ribs removed (from 2 stems)

Nonstick cooking spray

¼ cup grated Gruyère cheese

1 tablespoon shredded Parmesan

1. In a 2-cup measuring cup with a spout, whisk together the egg, milk, mustard, nutmeg, salt, and pepper. Add the bread and submerge it in the liquid.

2. Set the electric pressure cooker to the Sauté setting. When the pot is hot, pour in the avocado oil.

3. Add the onion, mushrooms, and thyme to the pot and sauté for 3 to 5 minutes or until the onion begins to soften. Stir in the kale and cook for about 2 minutes or until it wilts. Hit Cancel.

4. Spray the ramekins with cooking spray. Divide the mushroom mixture between the ramekins. Top each with 2 tablespoons Gruyère. Pour half of the egg mixture into each ramekin and stir. Make sure the bread stays submerged. Cover with foil.

5. Pour 1 cup of water into the electric pressure cooker and insert a wire rack or trivet. Place the ramekins on the rack.

6. Close and lock the lid of the pressure cooker. Set the valve to sealing.

7. Cook on high pressure for 8 minutes.

8. When the cooking is complete, hit Cancel. Allow the pressure to release naturally for 10 minutes, then quick release any remaining pressure.

9. Using tongs or the handles of the rack, transfer the ramekins to a cutting board. Carefully lift the foil and sprinkle the Parmesan on top. Replace the foil for about 5 minutes or until the cheese melts.

10. Remove the foil and serve immediately.

Ingredient tip: Do you miss bread and just don't like whole grain varieties? Try sourdough, which has a lower glycemic index than other white breads. You still need to watch the carbs, though.

PREP TIME:
5 minutes

COOK SETTING:
High

PRESSURE-UP
TIME: 21 minutes

COOK TIME:
35 minutes

RELEASE: Natural
for 20 minutes,
then Quick

TOTAL TIME:
1 hour 23 minutes

SPECIAL
EQUIPMENT:
kitchen twine

20-MINUTES-OR-
LESS PREP

GLUTEN FREE

VEGAN

FAMILY FRIENDLY

LOW SODIUM

PER SERVING
(½ CUP): Calories: 138;
Total Fat: 2g; Protein: 8g;
Carbohydrates: 23g;
Sugars: 4g; Fiber: 7g;
Sodium: 0mg

Salt-Free Chickpeas (Garbanzo Beans)

YIELD: 6 CUPS (23G CARBS PER SERVING)

I never considered cooking dried chickpeas until I read Patricia Wells' *Salad as a Meal*, where she says canned ones taste "tinny" and lack flavor. Since I first cooked my own, I've become a chickpea snob. Note that I haven't added any salt here; I prefer to season whatever dish I make that includes the cooked chickpeas. Save the cooking liquid (*aquafaba*) and use it as a substitute for egg whites in vegan meringue.

1 pound dried chickpeas

2 bay leaves

Fresh herbs, like parsley, thyme, rosemary, etc., cut into 3-inch pieces and tied together with kitchen twine (optional)

1. Rinse the chickpeas and put them in the electric pressure cooker. Add 8 cups of water, the bay leaves, and the herbs (if using).
2. Close and lock the lid. Turn the pressure valve to sealing.
3. Cook on high pressure for 35 minutes.
4. When the cooking is complete, hit Cancel. Allow the pressure to release naturally for 20 minutes, then quick release any remaining pressure.
5. Unlock and remove the lid. Discard the bay leaves and herb bundle.
6. Transfer the chickpeas to storage containers, covered with the cooking liquid, and let cool. Refrigerate for 3 or 4 days or freeze for up to 6 months.

Repurpose tip: Freeze cooked chickpeas in 1½-cup portions, and use them whenever a recipe calls for a 15-ounce can of chickpeas.

Stewed Chickpeas and Tomatoes

YIELD: 6 SERVINGS (35G CARBS PER SERVING)

Smoked paprika is the secret ingredient here; don't skip it. I wish I still had some of the Hungarian paprika my stepdaughter brought me after her semester in Budapest; it would be heavenly. Crushed tomatoes make for a smoother sauce, but diced or chopped can also be used.

2 tablespoons avocado oil

½ cup finely chopped onion

1 cup Vegetable Broth (page 116), divided

2 garlic cloves, minced

1 tablespoon smoked paprika

1 tablespoon tomato paste

1 (15-ounce) can crushed tomatoes

3 cups Salt-Free Chickpeas (page 58) or 2 (15-ounce) cans chickpeas, rinsed and drained

1 cup chopped lacinato kale leaves, stems and ribs removed (from 2 stems)

1. Set the electric pressure cooker to the Sauté setting. When the pot is hot, pour in the avocado oil.

2. Sauté the onion for 3 to 5 minutes or until it begins to soften. Stir in about 1 tablespoon of the broth, the garlic, paprika, and tomato paste. Hit Cancel.

3. Add the remaining broth, tomatoes, and chickpeas.

4. Close and lock the lid of the pressure cooker. Set the valve to sealing.

5. Cook on high pressure for 10 minutes.

6. When the cooking is complete, hit Cancel and allow the pressure to release naturally for 15 minutes, then quick release any remaining pressure.

7. Once the pin drops, unlock and remove the lid.

8. Stir in the kale and let everything sit in the pot for about 10 minutes or until the kale wilts.

9. Spoon into bowls and serve.

Ingredient tip: Lacinato kale (aka dinosaur kale) is not curly but has long slender leaves that are a blue-green color. I prefer it to other varieties because it's less bitter. You could also use spinach if you aren't a kale fan.

PREP TIME:
10 minutes

COOK SETTINGS:
Sauté, High

SAUTÉ TIME:
7 minutes

PRESSURE-UP TIME: 10 minutes

COOK TIME:
10 minutes

RELEASE: Natural for 15 minutes, then Quick

TOTAL TIME:
1 hour 3 minutes

20-MINUTES-OR-LESS PREP

GLUTEN FREE

LOW SODIUM

VEGAN

FAMILY FRIENDLY

PER SERVING
(⅔ **CUP**): Calories: 232; Total Fat: 7g; Protein: 10g; Carbohydrates: 35g; Sugars: 9g; Fiber: 10g; Sodium: 138mg

Cauliflower Chickpea Curry

SERVES 8 (21G CARBS PER SERVING)

PREP TIME:
12 minutes

COOK SETTINGS:
Sauté, High

SAUTÉ TIME:
7 minutes

PRESSURE-UP TIME: 21 minutes

COOK TIME:
3 minutes

RELEASE: Natural

RELEASE TIME:
30 minutes

FINISHING TIME:
5 minutes

TOTAL TIME:
1 hour 18 minutes

20-MINUTES-OR-LESS PREP

GLUTEN FREE

VEGAN

FAMILY FRIENDLY

**PER SERVING
(1 CUP):** Calories: 160;
Total Fat: 4; Protein: 5g;
Carbohydrates: 21g;
Sugars: 8g; Fiber: 5g;
Sodium: 292mg

The first time I tried this recipe, I used a frozen cauliflower-carrot-broccoli combination, and the broccoli got way overcooked. Since most frozen vegetable mixtures contain broccoli, I went with a bag of cauliflower and a bag of carrots instead. The list of ingredients may look long, but the dish comes together without much hands-on time.

2 tablespoons avocado oil

1 medium onion, chopped

1½ tablespoons minced garlic

1 tablespoon peeled and minced fresh ginger

1½ tablespoons Garam Masala (page 118)

1 teaspoon ground turmeric

½ teaspoon kosher salt

1 tablespoon tomato paste

1 cup Vegetable Broth (page 116) or water

1 cup light coconut milk

1 (15-ounce) can diced tomatoes

1 (15-ounce) bag frozen cauliflower florets

1 (15-ounce) bag frozen carrots

1½ cups Salt-Free Chickpeas (page 58)

2 cups baby spinach (optional)

2 tablespoons chopped fresh cilantro (optional)

Lime wedges, for serving

1. Set the electric pressure cooker to the Sauté setting. When the pot is hot, pour in the avocado oil.
2. Sauté the onion for 3 to 5 minutes, until it begins to soften.
3. Add the garlic, ginger, garam masala, turmeric, salt, and tomato paste. Stir for a minute or two until fragrant, then hit Cancel.
4. Stir in the broth, coconut milk, tomatoes and their juices, cauliflower, and carrots.
5. Close and lock the lid of the pressure cooker. Set the valve to sealing.
6. Cook on high pressure for 3 minutes.
7. When the cooking is complete, hit Cancel and allow the pressure to release naturally.
8. Once the pin drops, unlock and remove the lid.
9. Stir in the chickpeas and spinach (if using). Replace the lid for about 5 minutes or until the chickpeas warm up and the spinach wilts.
10. Garnish with cilantro (if using) and serve with a squeeze of fresh lime juice.

Substitution tip: Use low-sodium vegetable broth from a carton or can. Use canned chickpeas (rinsed and drained). If you don't want to make your own garam masala, you may be able to find it in the spice aisle in your grocery store.

Lentils with Carrots

SERVES 6 (24G CARBS PER SERVING)

Mom didn't know she liked lentils until she taste-tested this recipe for me. Originally, I had included some leftover cooked Herbed Whole Turkey Breast (page 79), but Mom said she thought the lentils would be just as good without the turkey. She was right. Use the more substantial brown or green lentils for this dish; they are sold in bags with other dried beans and are usually just marked "lentils."

2 tablespoons avocado oil

1 medium onion, chopped

3 celery stalks, chopped

1 teaspoon herbes de Provence

2 large carrots, chopped

2 cups Vegetable Broth (page 116) or water

1 cup dried brown or green lentils, rinsed and drained

Kosher salt

Freshly ground black pepper

1. Set the electric pressure cooker to the Sauté setting. When the pot is hot, pour in the avocado oil.

2. Sauté the onion and celery for 3 to 5 minutes, until the vegetables begin to soften. Stir in the herbes de Provence and carrots. Hit Cancel. Stir in the broth and lentils.

3. Close and lock the lid of the pressure cooker. Set the valve to sealing.

4. Cook on high pressure for 12 minutes.

5. When the cooking is complete, hit Cancel and allow the pressure to release naturally for 10 minutes, then quick release any remaining pressure.

6. Once the pin drops, unlock and remove the lid.

7. Season with salt and pepper, spoon into bowls, and serve.

Ingredient tip: Shop for lentils in an Indian, Bangladeshi, Pakistani, or any South Asian grocery store if you're lucky enough to have one nearby. The lentils available there are generally cheaper and of better quality than those you find at the supermarket.

PREP TIME: 15 minutes

COOK SETTINGS: Sauté, High

SAUTÉ TIME: 10 minutes

PRESSURE-UP TIME: 6 minutes

COOK TIME: 12 minutes

RELEASE: Natural for 10 minutes, then Quick

TOTAL TIME: 54 minutes

20-MINUTES-OR-LESS PREP

GLUTEN FREE

LOW SODIUM

VEGAN

FAMILY FRIENDLY

PER SERVING (⅔ **CUP):** Calories: 178; Total Fat: 5g; Protein: 9g; Carbohydrates: 24g; Sugars: 3g; Fiber: 11g; Sodium: 45mg

Split Pea Soup

SERVES 4 (52G CARBS PER SERVING)

PREP TIME:
8 minutes

COOK SETTING:
High

**PRESSURE-UP
TIME:** 16 minutes

COOK TIME:
15 minutes

RELEASE: Natural
for 10 minutes,
then Quick

TOTAL TIME:
50 minutes

20-MINUTES-OR-
LESS PREP

GLUTEN FREE

LOW SODIUM

VEGAN

FAMILY FRIENDLY

**PER SERVING
(1¼ CUPS):**
Calories: 284;
Total Fat: 1g; Protein: 19g;
Carbohydrates: 52g;
Sugars: 9g; Fiber: 21g;
Sodium: 60mg

I once took a what-has-more-carbs quiz at a diabetes support group meeting, and the comparison was between split pea soup and a grilled cheese sandwich. While the split pea soup won the carb count race, I'd still rather eat it than a grilled cheese. Split peas are loaded with fiber, protein, and iron. Grilled cheese sandwiches are full of fat, sodium, and cholesterol. Which would you rather put in your body?

1½ cups dried green split peas, rinsed and drained

4 cups Vegetable Broth (page 116) or water

2 celery stalks, chopped

1 medium onion, chopped

2 carrots, chopped

3 garlic cloves, minced

1 teaspoon herbes de Provence

1 teaspoon liquid smoke

Kosher salt

Freshly ground black pepper

Shredded carrot, for garnish (optional)

1. In the electric pressure cooker, combine the peas, broth, celery, onion, carrots, garlic, herbes de Provence, and liquid smoke.

2. Close and lock the lid of the pressure cooker. Set the valve to sealing.

3. Cook on high pressure for 15 minutes.

4. When the cooking is complete, hit Cancel and allow the pressure to release naturally for 10 minutes, then quick release any remaining pressure.

5. Once the pin drops, unlock and remove the lid.

6. Stir the soup and season with salt and pepper.

7. Spoon into serving bowls and sprinkle shredded carrots on top (if using).

Ingredient tip: Most split pea soup recipes include ham for a smoky flavor. This version includes liquid smoke instead, which I was surprised to learn is a vegan product. Liquid smoke is made from real smoke. Hardwoods are burned and the smoke is collected in condensers. The condensed smoke is then concentrated to produce a more intense flavor. Look for liquid smoke near the barbecue sauce in your grocery store.

Curried Black-Eyed Peas

SERVES 12 (31G CARBS PER SERVING)

Black-eyed peas are a staple in Southern households on January 1st. The idea is that eating them along with collard greens and cornbread will bring good luck and wealth in the new year. (You can, of course, eat black-eyed peas on other days, too.) The coconut water adds a touch of sweetness here, but you can also use additional broth or water instead. Any curry blend you happen to have will work just fine.

1 pound dried black-eyed peas, rinsed and drained

4 cups Vegetable Broth (page 116)

1 cup coconut water

1 cup chopped onion

4 large carrots, coarsely chopped

1½ tablespoons curry powder

1 tablespoon minced garlic

1 teaspoon peeled and minced fresh ginger

1 tablespoon extra-virgin olive oil

Kosher salt (optional)

Lime wedges, for serving

1. In the electric pressure cooker, combine the black-eyed peas, broth, coconut water, onion, carrots, curry powder, garlic, and ginger. Drizzle the olive oil over the top.
2. Close and lock the lid of the pressure cooker. Set the valve to sealing.
3. Cook on high pressure for 25 minutes.
4. When the cooking is complete, hit Cancel and allow the pressure to release naturally for 10 minutes, then quick release any remaining pressure.
5. Once the pin drops, unlock and remove the lid.
6. Season with salt (if using) and squeeze some fresh lime juice on each serving.

Leftover tip: For breakfast, serve leftover black-eyed peas with a poached or fried egg and some Spiced Tomato Ketchup (page 123).

PREP TIME:
15 minutes

COOK SETTING:
High

PRESSURE-UP TIME: 15 minutes

COOK TIME:
25 minutes

RELEASE: Natural for 10 minutes, then Quick

TOTAL TIME:
1 hour 7 minutes

20-MINUTES-OR-LESS PREP

GLUTEN FREE

VEGAN

FAMILY FRIENDLY

PER SERVING
(½ **CUP**): Calories: 112; Total Fat: 3g; Protein: 10g; Carbohydrates: 31g; Sugars: 6g; Fiber: 6g; Sodium: 670mg

Salt-Free No-Soak Beans

MAKES 6 CUPS (24G CARBS PER SERVING)

PREP TIME:
2 minutes

COOK SETTING:
High

**PRESSURE-UP
TIME:** 15 minutes

COOK TIME:
25 to 40 minutes

RELEASE: Natural
for 20 minutes,
then Quick

TOTAL TIME:
1 hour 2 minutes to
1 hour 17 minutes

20-MINUTES-OR-
LESS PREP

VEGAN

FAMILY FRIENDLY

LOW SODIUM

GLUTEN FREE

PER SERVING
(½ CUP): Calories: 141;
Total Fat: 2g; Protein: 8g;
Carbohydrates: 24g;
Sugars: 1g; Fiber: 6g;
Sodium: 5mg

Home-cooked beans taste so much better than their canned cousins, but the canned ones are so convenient, aren't they? Here's an easy way to cook dried beans that requires no soaking or other forethought. Plus, you can control the amount of sodium. I don't add any salt during the cooking process because it can make beans tough and I'd rather season whatever dish uses the cooked beans.

1 pound dried beans, rinsed (unsoaked)

5 cups Vegetable Broth (page 116), Chicken Bone Broth (page 117), or water

1 tablespoon extra-virgin olive oil

1. In the electric pressure cooker, combine the beans and broth. Drizzle the oil on top. (The oil will help control the foam produced by the cooking beans.)
2. Close and lock the lid of the pressure cooker. Set the valve to sealing.
3. *For black beans*, cook on high pressure for 25 minutes.
4. *For pinto beans, navy beans, or great northern beans*, cook on high pressure for 30 minutes.
5. *For cannellini beans*, cook on high pressure for 40 minutes.
6. When the cooking is complete, hit Cancel and allow the pressure to release naturally for 20 minutes, then quick release any remaining pressure.
7. Once the pin drops, unlock and remove the lid.
8. Let the beans cool, then pack them into containers and cover with the cooking liquid. Refrigerate for 3 to 5 days or freeze for up to 8 months.

Repurpose tip: As with Salt-Free Chickpeas (page 58), you can freeze your cooked beans in 1½-cup portions and use them whenever a recipe calls for a 15-ounce can of beans. Keep some in your refrigerator to add a quick boost of fiber to soups or salads.

Black Bean Chipotle Chili

SERVES 8 (45G CARBS PER SERVING)

Chipotle chiles are just smoked jalapeños. Here, you can get their great smoky flavor via chipotle chili powder. If you can't find it, just use regular chili powder. If you're watching sodium and don't want to cook your own salt-free black beans or make your own low-sodium vegetable broth, you may want to cut back on the added kosher salt.

2 tablespoons avocado oil

1 medium onion, chopped

1 tablespoon minced garlic

2 teaspoons kosher salt

½ teaspoon ground cumin

1 teaspoon chipotle chili powder

¼ teaspoon freshly ground black pepper

3 medium carrots, cut into ¼-inch-thick rounds

2 medium sweet potatoes, chopped (about 10 ounces)

1 (28-ounce) carton or can diced tomatoes

3 cups cooked Salt-Free No-Soak Beans (page 64)

1 cup Vegetable Broth (page 116) or water

10 ounces frozen corn

2 avocados, chopped just before serving

1. Set the electric pressure cooker to the Sauté setting. When the pot is hot, pour in the avocado oil.
2. Sauté the onion for 3 to 5 minutes, until it begins to soften. Hit Cancel.
3. Stir in the garlic, salt, cumin, chili powder, and pepper. Add the carrots and sweet potatoes and stir to coat with spices. Stir in the tomatoes and their juices, beans, and broth.
4. Close and lock the lid of the pressure cooker. Set the valve to sealing.
5. Cook on high pressure for 15 minutes.
6. While the chili is cooking, remove the corn from the freezer and pour it into a colander. Rinse with water to accelerate thawing. Let the corn sit in the colander.
7. When the cooking is complete, hit Cancel. Let the pressure release naturally for 10 minutes, then quick release any remaining pressure.
8. Once the pin drops, unlock and remove the lid.
9. Stir in the corn and let the chili sit for 5 minutes.
10. Spoon into serving bowls and serve topped with avocado.

Substitution tip: Use 2 (15-ounce) cans of rinsed and drained black beans instead of the Salt-Free No-Soak Black Beans. For extra kick, try a blend of cayenne and black pepper (like McCormick Hot Shot!®) instead of all black pepper.

PREP TIME:
20 minutes

COOK SETTINGS:
Sauté, High

SAUTÉ TIME:
5 minutes

PRESSURE-UP TIME: 18 minutes

COOK TIME:
15 minutes

RELEASE: Natural for 10 minutes, then Quick

TOTAL TIME:
1 hour 15 minutes

20-MINUTES-OR-LESS PREP

GLUTEN FREE

VEGAN

FAMILY FRIENDLY

PER SERVING (1⅛ CUPS):
Calories: 295;
Total Fat: 10g; Protein: 10g;
Carbohydrates: 45g;
Sugars: 8g; Fiber: 11g;
Sodium: 723mg

PREP TIME:
16 minutes

COOK SETTING:
High

**PRESSURE-UP
TIME:** 15 minutes

COOK TIME:
7 minutes

RELEASE: Quick

TOTAL TIME:
35 minutes

**SPECIAL
EQUIPMENT:**
immersion blender

20-MINUTES-OR-
LESS PREP

GLUTEN FREE

VEGAN

FAMILY FRIENDLY

**PER SERVING
(1 CUP):** Calories: 196;
Total Fat: 6g; Protein: 7g;
Carbohydrates: 31g;
Sugars: 4g; Fiber: 8g;
Sodium: 332mg

Butternut Squash Stew
with White Beans

SERVES 6 (31G CARBS PER SERVING)

The hardest part of this recipe is peeling and seeding the squash. To save yourself some time, look for precut butternut squash in the produce section or in the freezer aisle of your grocery store. I prefer smaller white beans, but cannellinis will work, too. If you like things spicy, use a hotter fresh chile, like a jalapeño or serrano, to replace the poblano. If you're hard-core, try a ghost pepper or habanero.

1 pound butternut squash, peeled, seeded, and cut into 1-inch cubes (about 3 cups)

1 tablespoon extra-virgin olive oil

1 tablespoon chili powder

1 teaspoon dried oregano

1 teaspoon ground cumin

1 tablespoon garlic pepper or garlic powder

½ teaspoon kosher salt

2 tablespoons finely chopped poblano chile or green bell pepper

3 cups Vegetable Broth (page 116) or water

1 (15-ounce) can diced tomatoes

1 (15-ounce) can white beans, rinsed and drained

1 avocado, chopped just before serving

1. In the electric pressure cooker, toss the squash with the olive oil, chili powder, oregano, cumin, garlic pepper, and salt.
2. Stir in the poblano, broth, and tomatoes and their juices.
3. Close and lock the lid of the pressure cooker. Set the valve to sealing.
4. Cook on high pressure for 7 minutes.
5. When the cooking is complete, hit Cancel and quick release the pressure.
6. Once the pin drops, unlock and remove the lid.
7. Stir in the beans and let the stew sit for about 5 minutes to let the beans warm up.
8. Use an immersion blender to purée about one-third of the stew right in the pot. (I like to leave some chunks of squash and whole beans for more texture.)
9. Spoon into serving bowls and top with the avocado.

Make-ahead tip: Complete the stew through step 6, cool it, and refrigerate. When you're ready to eat, purée about one-third of the stew and some of the beans in a food processor or blender. Combine the puréed mixture with the remaining stew and beans in a saucepan, and warm it up on the stovetop. Spoon into serving bowls and top with the avocado.

15-Bean Pistou Soup

SERVES 6 (34G CARBS PER SERVING)

Pistou is a condiment used in the Provence region of France that is similar to pesto. It is most often served atop thick vegetable soups, especially those made with the fresh beans abundant there in the summer. Since fresh beans are harder to come by in the United States, I've made a simpler version of pistou soup using dried beans and pesto that can be enjoyed any time of the year.

10 ounces 15-Bean Soup mix, beans only, rinsed and drained (half of a 20-ounce bag)

4 cups Vegetable Broth (page 116) or water

½ cup chopped onion

½ cup chopped green bell pepper

1 celery stalk, chopped

1 tablespoon minced garlic

½ teaspoon Italian seasoning

1 bay leaf

1 tablespoon extra-virgin olive oil

2 tablespoons tomato paste

6 tablespoons 5-Minute Pesto (page 119) or store-bought pesto

PREP TIME:
12 minutes

COOK SETTINGS:
High, Sauté

PRESSURE-UP TIME: 14 minutes

COOK TIME:
45 minutes

RELEASE: Natural for 20 minutes, then Quick

TOTAL TIME:
1 hour 36 minutes

20-MINUTES-OR-LESS PREP

GLUTEN FREE

FAMILY FRIENDLY

LOW SODIUM

PER SERVING
(1 CUP): Calories: 292; Total Fat: 13g; Protein: 13g; Carbohydrates: 34g; Sugars: 3g; Fiber: 8g; Sodium: 125mg

1. In the electric pressure cooker, combine the beans, broth, onion, bell pepper, celery, garlic, Italian seasoning, and bay leaf. Drizzle the olive oil over the top. (The oil will help control the foam produced by the cooking beans.)

2. Close and lock the lid of the pressure cooker. Set the valve to sealing.

3. Cook on high pressure for 45 minutes.

4. When the cooking is complete, hit Cancel. Allow the pressure to release naturally for 20 minutes, then quick release any remaining pressure.

5. Once the pin drops, unlock and remove the lid.

6. Stir in the tomato paste and hit Sauté. Cook for about 5 minutes or until the soup thickens. Discard the bay leaf.

7. Spoon into serving bowls and top each with 1 tablespoon of pesto.

Ingredient tip: The 15-Bean Soup is a mixture of dried legumes that includes a packet of seasoning mix. It can usually be found near the other dried beans in your grocery store and includes pinto beans, black-eyed peas, cranberry beans, split peas, and lentils. In this recipe, you will use the beans but not the seasoning packet. If you can't find 15-Bean Soup, mix up any combination of your favorite dried legumes instead.

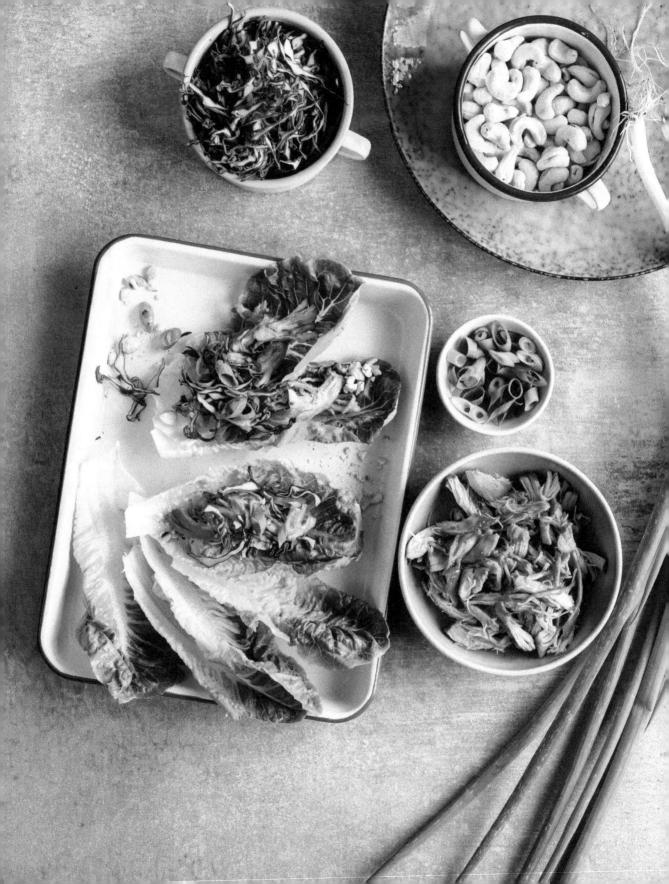

5

Poultry

PREP TIME:
20 minutes

COOK SETTING:
High

**PRESSURE-UP
TIME:** 20 minutes

COOK TIME:
21 minutes

RELEASE: Natural
for 15 minutes,
then Quick

TOTAL TIME:
1 hour 16 minutes

20-MINUTES-OR-
LESS PREP

GLUTEN FREE

LOW CARB

FAMILY FRIENDLY

PER SERVING:
Calories: 215;
Total Fat: 9g; Protein: 25g;
Carbohydrates: 5g;
Sugars: 2g; Fiber: 1g;
Sodium: 847mg

Smoky Whole Chicken

SERVES 6 (5G CARBS PER SERVING)

Cooking a whole chicken in your EPC is almost as easy as buying a precooked rotisserie chicken. You'll get great flavor and juiciness by stuffing lemons in the cavity and including some smoky paprika. The rule of thumb for cooking whole chickens is 6 minutes per pound: a 3-pound chicken will take 18 minutes, and a 4-pound chicken will take 24 minutes. Make sure to eat the cooked garlic, too!

2 tablespoons extra-virgin olive oil

1 tablespoon kosher salt

1½ teaspoons smoked paprika

1 teaspoon freshly ground
black pepper

½ teaspoon herbes de Provence

¼ teaspoon cayenne pepper

1 (3½-pound) whole chicken, rinsed
and patted dry, giblets removed

1 large lemon, halved

6 garlic cloves, peeled and crushed
with the flat side of a knife

1 large onion, cut into
8 wedges, divided

1 cup Chicken Bone Broth (page 117),
low-sodium store-bought chicken
broth, or water

2 large carrots, each cut into 4 pieces

2 celery stalks, each cut into 4 pieces

1. In a small bowl, combine the olive oil, salt, paprika, pepper, herbes de Provence, and cayenne.

2. Place the chicken on a cutting board and rub the olive oil mixture under the skin and all over the outside. Stuff the cavity with the lemon halves, garlic cloves, and 3 to 4 wedges of onion.

3. Pour the broth into the electric pressure cooker. Add the remaining onion wedges, carrots, and celery. Insert a wire rack or trivet on top of the vegetables.

4. Place the chicken, breast-side up, on the rack.

5. Close and lock the lid of the pressure cooker. Set the valve to sealing.

6. Cook on high pressure for 21 minutes.

7. When the cooking is complete, hit Cancel and allow the pressure to release naturally for 15 minutes, then quick release any remaining pressure.

8. Once the pin drops, unlock and remove the lid.

9. Carefully remove the chicken to a clean cutting board. Remove the skin and cut the chicken into pieces or shred/chop the meat, and serve.

Repurpose tip: Save the bones to make Chicken Bone Broth (page 117, and strain the liquid remaining in the pot to replace some of the water in the bone broth recipe for even more flavor.

Firecracker Chicken Meatballs

SERVES 6 (17G CARBS PER SERVING)

PREP TIME:
15 minutes

COOK SETTINGS:
Sauté, High

SAUTÉ TIME:
15 minutes

**PRESSURE-UP
TIME:** 8 minutes

COOK TIME:
6 minutes

RELEASE: Natural
for 10 minutes,
then Quick

TOTAL TIME:
55 minutes

20-MINUTES-OR-
LESS PREP

FAMILY FRIENDLY

**PER SERVING
(5 MEATBALLS):**
Calories: 244;
Total Fat: 12g; Protein: 18g;
Carbohydrates: 17g;
Sugars: 7g; Fiber: 2g;
Sodium: 989mg

These spicy meatballs certainly live up to their name, and they are the perfect game-watching snack. Serve them with raw carrot and celery sticks and lower-fat blue cheese or ranch dressing on the side. Feel free to make larger meatballs, but note that they may take longer to cook.

For the sauce

½ cup hot sauce (such as Frank's RedHot)

2 tablespoons honey

2 tablespoons low-sodium soy sauce or tamari

For the meatballs

1 pound ground chicken or turkey

1 cup Panko breadcrumbs (whole wheat, if possible)

1 large egg, slightly beaten

1½ teaspoons garlic pepper

1 teaspoon onion powder

¼ teaspoon kosher salt

2 tablespoons avocado oil, divided

To make the sauce

In a 1-cup measuring cup, whisk together the hot sauce, honey, and soy sauce.

To make the meatballs

1. In a large bowl, combine the chicken, Panko, egg, garlic pepper, onion powder, and salt. Mix gently with your hands until just combined. (Do not overmix or your meatballs will be tough.)

2. Pinch off about a tablespoon of the meat mixture and roll it into a ball. (A 1½-inch cookie scoop makes the job easy.) Repeat with the remaining meat. You should end up with about 30 (1½-inch) meatballs.

3. Set the electric pressure cooker to the Sauté/More setting. When the pot is hot, pour in 1 tablespoon of avocado oil.

4. Add half of the meatballs around the edge of the pot and brown them for 3 to 5 minutes. (The oil tends to pool towards the outside of the pot, so the meatballs will get browner if you put them there. Leaving space in the middle of the pot will also make it easier to turn the meatballs.) Flip the meatballs over and brown the other side for 3 to 5 minutes. Transfer to a paper towel–lined plate and repeat with the remaining 1 tablespoon of avocado oil and meatballs. Hit Cancel.

5. Return the meatballs to the pot and pour in the sauce mixture. Stir to coat all sides of the meatballs with sauce, then arrange them in a single layer.

6. Close and lock the lid of the pressure cooker. Set the valve to sealing.

7. Cook on high pressure for 6 minutes.

8. When the cooking is complete, hit Cancel. Allow the pressure to release naturally for 10 minutes, then quick release any remaining pressure.

9. Once the pin drops, unlock and remove the lid. Stir to evenly distribute the sauce.

10. Serve with toothpicks as an appetizer or as a main dish.

Make-ahead tip: Complete steps 1 through 4, let the meatballs cool, and freeze them. When you are ready to eat, make the sauce and then jump to step 5, using the frozen meatballs.

Chicken Salsa Verde with Pumpkin

SERVES 4 (13G CARBS PER SERVING)

PREP TIME:
10 minutes

COOK SETTINGS:
Sauté, High

SAUTÉ TIME:
5 minutes

PRESSURE-UP TIME: 9 minutes

COOK TIME:
5 minutes

RELEASE: Quick

TOTAL TIME:
30 minutes

20-MINUTES-OR-LESS PREP

GLUTEN FREE

FAMILY FRIENDLY

PER SERVING
(1 CUP): Calories: 238;
Total Fat: 10g; Protein: 23g;
Carbohydrates: 13g;
Sugars: 5g; Fiber: 4g;
Sodium: 407mg

Do you need a way to use up leftover chicken? Try this quick stew featuring green salsa and pumpkin for a boost of vitamin A. Be careful not to buy pumpkin pie filling (which is sweetened)—you want 100 percent pumpkin for this recipe. If you prefer a vegan option, substitute white beans for the chicken and use vegetable broth instead of bone broth.

2 tablespoons avocado oil

1 small onion, chopped

½ tablespoon dried oregano

3 garlic cloves, finely minced

1 cup Chicken Bone Broth (page 117) or Vegetable Broth (page 116)

¾ cup canned pumpkin purée

1 cup Roasted Tomatillo Salsa (page 121) or salsa verde

2 cups shredded cooked chicken breast

Thinly sliced jalapeño chiles, for garnish (optional)

Chopped fresh cilantro, for garnish (optional)

1. Set the electric pressure cooker to the Sauté setting. When the pot is hot, pour in the avocado oil.
2. Sauté the onion for 3 to 5 minutes or until it begins to soften. Hit Cancel.
3. Stir in the oregano, garlic, broth, pumpkin, salsa, and chicken.
4. Close and lock the lid of the pressure cooker. Set the valve to sealing.
5. Cook on high pressure for 5 minutes.
6. When the cooking is complete, hit Cancel and quick release the pressure.
7. Once the pin drops, unlock and remove the lid.
8. Spoon into serving bowls and garnish with jalapeños and cilantro (if using).

Ingredient tip: Salsa verde is made with tomatillos instead of tomatoes, and is green instead of red. You'll find it bottled or canned in various heat levels. If you're watching sodium, make your own Roasted Tomatillo Salsa (page 121) so you can control the amount of salt.

Shredded Buffalo Chicken

SERVES 8 (2G CARBS PER SERVING)

Do you love spicy chicken wings? This EPC version of Buffalo chicken gives you all of the same flavors with much less fat and mess. This dish is great when you cook for folks who complain about eating "healthy" food. You can serve your chicken on top of a salad (try it with blue cheese dressing made with yogurt!), and they can have theirs in a quesadilla or on top of a baked potato.

2 tablespoons avocado oil

½ cup finely chopped onion

1 celery stalk, finely chopped

1 large carrot, chopped

⅓ cup mild hot sauce (such as Frank's RedHot)

½ tablespoon apple cider vinegar

¼ teaspoon garlic powder

2 bone-in, skin-on chicken breasts (about 2 pounds)

1. Set the electric pressure cooker to the Sauté setting. When the pot is hot, pour in the avocado oil.

2. Sauté the onion, celery, and carrot for 3 to 5 minutes or until the onion begins to soften. Hit Cancel.

3. Stir in the hot sauce, vinegar, and garlic powder. Place the chicken breasts in the sauce, meat-side down.

4. Close and lock the lid of the pressure cooker. Set the valve to sealing.

5. Cook on high pressure for 20 minutes.

6. When cooking is complete, hit Cancel and quick release the pressure. Once the pin drops, unlock and remove the lid.

7. Using tongs, transfer the chicken breasts to a cutting board. When the chicken is cool enough to handle, remove the skin, shred the chicken and return it to the pot. Let the chicken soak in the sauce for at least 5 minutes.

8. Serve immediately.

Make-ahead tip: Cook the chicken, then let it cool and refrigerate it. It will keep for 3 to 4 days. Use the chicken in salads, quesadillas, lettuce wraps, burritos, nachos, tacos, or on top of baked potatoes.

PREP TIME:
10 minutes

COOK SETTINGS:
Sauté, High

SAUTÉ TIME:
7 minutes

PRESSURE-UP TIME: 9 minutes

COOK TIME:
20 minutes

RELEASE: Quick

TOTAL TIME:
58 minutes

20-MINUTES-OR-LESS PREP

GLUTEN FREE

LOW CARB

FAMILY FRIENDLY

PER SERVING
(½ **CUP**): Calories: 139; Total Fat: 9g; Protein: 12g; Carbohydrates: 2g; Sugars: 1g; Fiber: 1g; Sodium: 295mg

PREP TIME:
20 minutes

COOK SETTINGS:
High, Sauté

**PRESSURE-UP
TIME:** 15 minutes

COOK TIME:
20 minutes

RELEASE: Natural for
5 minutes, then Quick

TOTAL TIME:
1 hour 20 minutes

20-MINUTES-OR-
LESS PREP

LOW SODIUM

**PER SERVING
(½ CUP CHICKEN,
PLUS ½ CUP SLAW):**
Calories: 203;
Total Fat: 9g; Protein: 13g;
Carbohydrates: 16g;
Sugars: 12g; Fiber: 2g;
Sodium: 80mg

Beer-Braised Chicken with Grape-Apple Slaw

SERVES 8 (16G CARBS PER SERVING)

Many dishes cooked in the EPC don't have a tremendous amount of color. This one features a fresh slaw with purple cabbage, green grapes, and red and white apples. If you know more about beer than I do, pick an ale that will complement the fruit in the slaw. The prep time sounds long, but it overlaps with the cook time. Don't forget to save the bones for making Chicken Bone Broth (page 117).

For the chicken

1 cup brown ale

1 teaspoon white wheat flour

2 bone-in, skin-on chicken breasts (about 2 pounds)

Kosher salt

Freshly ground black pepper

1 tablespoon coarse-grain mustard

For the slaw

¼ cup cider vinegar

2 tablespoons extra-virgin olive oil

1 tablespoon honey

1 tablespoon coarse-grain mustard

Kosher salt

Freshly ground black pepper

¼ head purple or red cabbage, thinly sliced

2 cups seedless green grapes, halved

1 medium apple, cut into matchstick-size slices (I like Gala)

To make the chicken

1. In a 2-cup measuring cup or small bowl, whisk together the ale and flour. Pour into the electric pressure cooker.

2. Sprinkle the chicken breasts with salt and pepper. Place them in the electric pressure cooker, meat-side down.

3. Close and lock the lid of the pressure cooker. Set the valve to sealing.

4. Cook on high pressure for 20 minutes. While the chicken is cooking, make the slaw.

5. When the cooking is complete, hit Cancel. Allow the pressure to release naturally for 5 minutes, then quick release any remaining pressure.

6. Once the pin drops, unlock and remove the lid.

7. Using tongs, remove the chicken breasts to a cutting board. Hit Sauté/More and bring the liquid in the pot to a boil, scraping up any brown bits on the bottom of the pot. Cook, stirring occasionally, for about 5 minutes or until the sauce has reduced in volume by about a third. Hit Cancel and whisk in the mustard.

8. When the chicken is cool enough to handle, remove the skin, shred the meat, and return it to the pot. Let the chicken soak in the sauce for at least 5 minutes.

9. Serve the chicken topped with the slaw.

To make the slaw

1. In a small jar with a screw-top lid, combine the vinegar, olive oil, honey, and mustard. Shake well, then season with salt and pepper, and shake again.

2. In a large bowl, toss together the cabbage, grapes, and apple. Add the dressing and mix well. Let the mixture sit at room temperature while the chicken cooks.

Make-ahead tip: Make the slaw ahead of time and refrigerate. The slaw will only get better as it sits. Stir well before serving.

Teriyaki Chicken

SERVES 4 (9G CARBS PER SERVING)

PREP TIME:
10 minutes

COOK SETTINGS:
High, Sauté

**PRESSURE-UP
TIME:** 10 minutes

COOK TIME:
15 minutes

RELEASE: Quick

TOTAL TIME:
42 minutes

20-MINUTES-OR-
LESS PREP

GLUTEN FREE

LOW CARB

FAMILY FRIENDLY

PER SERVING:
Calories: 214;
Total Fat: 6g; Protein: 30g;
Carbohydrates: 9g;
Sugars: 6g; Fiber: 1g;
Sodium: 540mg

I much prefer the texture of boneless chicken thighs cooked in the EPC to boneless chicken breasts, but thighs are higher in fat and calories. It's worth the splurge here. Serve this chicken with riced cauliflower or a small portion of brown rice and stir-fried vegetables. Frozen cauliflower and vegetables can be microwaved quickly for easy sides—no chopping required.

3 tablespoons low-sodium gluten-free tamari or soy sauce

¼ cup canned crushed pineapple

2 tablespoons dark brown sugar

2 tablespoons minced garlic

1 tablespoon peeled and minced fresh ginger

2 scallions, both white and green parts, thinly sliced, divided

1½ pounds boneless, skinless chicken thighs

Sesame seeds, for garnish

1. In the electric pressure cooker, combine the tamari, pineapple, brown sugar, garlic, ginger, and white parts of the scallions. Dip the chicken thighs in the sauce to coat all sides, then nestle each piece in the sauce in a single layer.

2. Close and lock the lid of the pressure cooker. Set the valve to sealing.

3. Cook on high pressure for 15 minutes.

4. When the cooking is complete, hit Cancel and quick release the pressure.

5. Once the pin drops, unlock and remove the lid.

6. Hit Sauté and simmer until the sauce has thickened and is the consistency you like, about 5 minutes. Hit Cancel. Shred or chop the chicken, if desired.

7. Remove the chicken to serving plates or a platter, sprinkle with the green parts of the scallions and sesame seeds. Serve immediately.

Substitution tip: Use ¾ cup of bottled teriyaki sauce instead of the soy sauce, pineapple, brown sugar, garlic, and ginger. Pick the brand that is lowest in sodium and sugar.

Herbed Whole Turkey Breast

SERVES 12 (0G CARBS PER SERVING)

Bone-in turkey breast is so tender and juicy when cooked in the EPC. The rule of thumb for cooking time is 5 minutes per pound, so a 5-pounder would need 25 minutes, a 6-pounder would need 30 minutes, and a 7-pounder would need 35 minutes. Before you start, make sure the turkey breast fits in your EPC (along with the rack). A 6-pound breast fits fine in my 6-quart EPC.

3 tablespoons extra-virgin olive oil

1½ tablespoons herbes de Provence or poultry seasoning

2 teaspoons minced garlic

1 teaspoon lemon zest (from 1 small lemon)

1 tablespoon kosher salt

1½ teaspoons freshly ground black pepper

1 (6-pound) bone-in, skin-on whole turkey breast, rinsed and patted dry

1. In a small bowl, whisk together the olive oil, herbes de Provence, garlic, lemon zest, salt, and pepper.
2. Rub the outside of the turkey and under the skin with the olive oil mixture.
3. Pour 1 cup of water into the electric pressure cooker and insert a wire rack or trivet.
4. Place the turkey on the rack, skin-side up.
5. Close and lock the lid of the pressure cooker. Set the valve to sealing.
6. Cook on high pressure for 30 minutes.
7. When the cooking is complete, hit Cancel. Allow the pressure to release naturally for 20 minutes, then quick release any remaining pressure.
8. Once the pin drops, unlock and remove the lid.
9. Carefully transfer the turkey to a cutting board. Remove the skin, slice, and serve.

Leftover tip: Use leftover turkey on top of salads, in tacos, or in any recipe that calls for cooked chicken. Try adding some chopped turkey to Lentils with Carrots (page 61). Save the bones to make Chicken Bone Broth (page 117).

PREP TIME:
10 minutes

COOK SETTING:
High

PRESSURE-UP TIME: 17 minutes

COOK TIME:
30 minutes

RELEASE: Natural for 20 minutes, then Quick

TOTAL TIME:
1 hour 17 minutes

20-MINUTES-OR-LESS PREP

GLUTEN FREE

LOW CARB

SUGAR FREE

FAMILY FRIENDLY

PER SERVING:
Calories: 146;
Total Fat: 9g; Protein: 16g;
Carbohydrates: 0g;
Sugars: 0g; Fiber: 0g;
Sodium: 413mg

Hoisin Chicken Lettuce Wraps

SERVES 4 (18G CARBS PER SERVING)

PREP TIME:
10 minutes

COOK SETTING:
High

**PRESSURE-UP
TIME:** 8 minutes

COOK TIME:
20 minutes

RELEASE: Quick

TOTAL TIME:
45 minutes

20-MINUTES-OR-
LESS PREP

GLUTEN FREE

FAMILY FRIENDLY

PER SERVING:
Calories: 233;
Total Fat: 13g; Protein: 14g;
Carbohydrates: 18g;
Sugars: 10g; Fiber: 2g;
Sodium: 1080mg

Hoisin sauce makes for some tasty Chinese food, but it's incredibly high in sodium. Here, I've tried to recreate the flavors with a bit less salt. The chicken breast is cooked, then served in lettuce cups with broccoli slaw and cashews for crunch. Who needs rice? The Sriracha gives the sauce some punch. If you don't like things too spicy, simply leave it out.

For the chicken

2 teaspoons peanut oil

⅓ cup low-sodium gluten-free tamari or soy sauce

1 tablespoon honey

2 tablespoons rice vinegar

2 teaspoons Sriracha sauce

1 tablespoon minced garlic

2 teaspoons peeled and minced fresh ginger

⅓ cup Chicken Bone Broth (page 117) or water

2 scallions, both white and green parts, thinly sliced, divided

1 bone-in, skin-on chicken breast (about 1 pound)

For the lettuce wraps

Large lettuce leaves (preferably Bibb)

1 cup broccoli slaw or shredded cabbage

¼ cup chopped cashews, toasted (see page 120)

To make the chicken

1. In the electric pressure cooker, whisk together the peanut oil, tamari, honey, rice vinegar, Sriracha, garlic, ginger, and broth. Stir in the white parts of the scallions.

2. Place the chicken breast in the sauce, meat-side down.

3. Close and lock the lid of the pressure cooker. Set the valve to sealing.

4. Cook on high pressure for 20 minutes.

5. When the cooking is complete, hit Cancel and quick release the pressure.

6. Once the pin drops, unlock and remove the lid.

7. Using tongs, transfer the chicken breast to a cutting board. When the chicken is cool enough to handle, remove the skin, shred the chicken, and return it to the pot. Let the chicken soak in the sauce for at least 5 minutes.

To make the lettuce wraps

1. Spoon some of the chicken and sauce into the lettuce leaves.

2. Sprinkle with the broccoli slaw, the green parts of the scallions, and the cashews.

3. Serve immediately.

Make-ahead tip: Cook the chicken through step 6, then cool and refrigerate both the chicken breast and the sauce. When you are ready to eat, remove the skin, shred the meat, heat up the chicken and sauce (if desired), and assemble the lettuce wraps.

SERVES 6 (3G CARBS PER SERVING)

PREP TIME:
5 minutes

COOK SETTING:
High

**PRESSURE-UP
TIME:** 13 minutes

COOK TIME:
8 minutes

RELEASE: Natural
for 10 minutes,
then Quick

TOTAL TIME:
36 minutes

20-MINUTES-OR-
LESS PREP

GLUTEN FREE

LOW CARB

FAMILY FRIENDLY

PER SERVING:
Calories: 168;
Total Fat: 5g; Protein: 28g;
Carbohydrates: 3g;
Sugars: 2g; Fiber: 1g;
Sodium: 559mg

Unseasoned turkey tenderloin can sometimes be hard to find. If your store only has the seasoned ones, rinse off all of the seasoning (to get rid of as much sodium as possible), then pat the tenderloins dry with paper towels. You can also use pork tenderloin or chicken instead. Try a Mexican cheese blend that contains Monterey Jack, Colby, and cheddar.

1 cup Low-Sodium Salsa (page 122) or bottled salsa

1 teaspoon chili powder

½ teaspoon ground cumin

¼ teaspoon dried oregano

1½ pounds unseasoned turkey tenderloin or boneless turkey breast, cut into 6 pieces

Freshly ground black pepper

½ cup shredded Monterey Jack cheese or Mexican cheese blend

1. In a small bowl or measuring cup, combine the salsa, chili powder, cumin, and oregano. Pour half of the mixture into the electric pressure cooker.
2. Nestle the turkey into the sauce. Grind some pepper onto each piece of turkey. Pour the remaining salsa mixture on top.
3. Close and lock the lid of the pressure cooker. Set the valve to sealing.
4. Cook on high pressure for 8 minutes.
5. When the cooking is complete, hit Cancel. Allow the pressure to release naturally for 10 minutes, then quick release any remaining pressure.
6. Once the pin drops, unlock and remove the lid.
7. Sprinkle the cheese on top, and put the lid back on for a few minutes to let the cheese melt.
8. Serve immediately.

Substitution tip: Use any type of salsa or picante sauce you like. Try to buy a brand that's low in sodium.

Sausage and Cauliflower "Grits"

SERVES 4 (11G CARBS PER SERVING)

This dish isn't very colorful, but it more than makes up for that in flavor. My husband discovered chicken sausage with kale on a shopping trip, and it was fantastic in this recipe. And who doesn't need more leafy greens in their diet? Riced cauliflower makes a great substitute for higher-carb corn grits. (Hit the unopened bag of frozen cauliflower on the edge of your kitchen counter a few times to break up any clumps.)

1 pound frozen (uncooked) Italian-style chicken or turkey sausages

1 pound frozen riced cauliflower, broken up

1 tablespoon extra-virgin olive oil

Freshly ground black pepper

⅓ cup shredded Parmesan cheese

Chopped fresh parsley, for garnish

1. Pour ½ cup of water into the electric pressure cooker and add the sausages.
2. Close and lock the lid of the pressure cooker. Set the valve to sealing.
3. Cook on high pressure for 15 minutes.
4. When the cooking is complete, hit Cancel and quick release the pressure.
5. Once the pin drops, unlock and remove the lid.
6. Using tongs, transfer the sausages to a cutting board and slice into 1-inch rounds. Pour the liquid from the pot into a measuring cup. Pour ½ cup of the liquid back into the pot; discard the rest.
7. In the electric pressure cooker, combine the sliced sausage, cauliflower, olive oil, and pepper. Close and lock the lid of the pressure cooker. Set the valve to sealing.
8. Cook on high pressure for 5 minutes.
9. When the cooking is complete, hit Cancel and quick release the pressure.
10. Once the pin drops, unlock and remove the lid.
11. Stir in the Parmesan, garnish with parsley, and serve immediately.

Substitution tip: If you want to use precooked chicken sausage to save yourself some time, skip steps 1 through 5 and add ½ cup of Chicken Bone Broth (page 117) along with the other ingredients in step 6.

PREP TIME:
7 minutes

COOK SETTING:
High

PRESSURE-UP TIME: 22 minutes

COOK TIME:
20 minutes

RELEASE: Quick

TOTAL TIME:
52 minutes

20-MINUTES-OR-LESS PREP

FAMILY FRIENDLY

PER SERVING:
Calories: 263;
Total Fat: 11g; Protein: 30g;
Carbohydrates: 11g;
Sugars: 4g; Fiber: 3g;
Sodium: 660mg

Spaghetti and Turkey Meatballs

SERVES 6 (45G CARBS PER SERVING)

PREP TIME:
5 minutes

COOK SETTING:
High

PRESSURE-UP TIME: 19 minutes

COOK TIME:
10 minutes

RELEASE: Quick

TOTAL TIME:
37 minutes

20-MINUTES-OR-LESS PREP

FAMILY FRIENDLY

PER SERVING:
Calories: 479;
Total Fat: 21g; Protein: 31g;
Carbohydrates: 45g;
Sugars: 8g; Fiber: 7g;
Sodium: 1237mg

This is the perfect example of how to make a meal that satisfies the pasta lovers in the family and can be easily adapted for a diabetes-friendly diet. Make the recipe, then set aside some meatballs for the low-carb folks to serve with "zoodles" (noodles made from zucchini). Everyone gets what they need. But moreover, I love that you can cook noodles, sauce, and meatballs in one pot.

1 recipe (about 22) frozen Italian Turkey Sausage Meatballs (page 125)

8 ounces whole grain thin spaghetti (uncooked), broken in half

1 tablespoon extra-virgin olive oil

1 (24-ounce) jar pasta sauce or 3 cups homemade sauce

Freshly grated Parmesan cheese, for serving (optional)

1. In the electric pressure cooker, arrange the frozen meatballs in a single layer. (Depending on the size of your meatballs and the size of your EPC, you may need more or less than 22.)

2. Place the broken spaghetti on top of the meatballs in an even layer. Drizzle the olive oil all over the spaghetti.

3. Pour in 3 cups of water and the pasta sauce. If the spaghetti is not completely covered, add a bit more water. Do not stir.

4. Close and lock the lid of the pressure cooker. Set the valve to sealing.

5. Cook on high pressure for 10 minutes.

6. When the cooking is complete, hit Cancel and quick release the pressure.

7. Once the pin drops, unlock and remove the lid.

8. Serve with Parmesan cheese (if using).

Substitution tip: Feel free to use other frozen meatballs if you don't want to make your own. Look for chicken or turkey instead of meat, and pick the brand that is lowest in fat, sodium, and carbs.

Okra Stew with Chicken Andouille Sausage and Shrimp

SERVES 4 (24G CARBS PER SERVING)

PREP TIME:
10 minutes

COOK SETTINGS:
Sauté, High

SAUTÉ TIME:
10 minutes

PRESSURE-UP TIME: 10 minutes

COOK TIME:
20 minutes

RELEASE: Quick

TOTAL TIME:
57 minutes

20-MINUTES-OR-LESS PREP

GLUTEN FREE

FAMILY FRIENDLY

PER SERVING (1¼ CUPS):
Calories: 252;
Total Fat: 12g; Protein: 16g;
Carbohydrates: 24g;
Sugars: 10g; Fiber: 6g;
Sodium: 732mg

Okra may not be the miracle cure for diabetes you've read about, but it does contain soluble fiber that slows down the rate at which glucose enters the bloodstream. If you think you don't like okra, try this stew. The okra dissolves and fools you into thinking it's green pepper instead. It also thickens the stew, so you don't need any flour. Prefer a vegan option? Skip the sausage and shrimp.

3 tablespoons avocado oil, divided

½ large onion, halved and then cut into ¼-inch-thick slices

8 ounces okra, cut into ½-inch-thick slices

¼ teaspoon kosher salt

¼ teaspoon freshly ground black pepper

3 garlic cloves, minced

1 teaspoon dried oregano

1 (28-ounce) carton or can chopped tomatoes

2 links precooked chicken andouille sausage, cut into ¼-inch-thick slices (about 6 ounces)

8 ounces raw shrimp (26 to 35 count), peeled and deveined

Fresh parsley, chopped

1. Set the electric pressure cooker to the Sauté setting. When the pot is hot, pour in 1½ tablespoons avocado oil.

2. Add the onion and sauté for 3 to 5 minutes or until it begins to soften.

3. Add the remaining 1½ tablespoons olive oil and okra to the pot. Sprinkle with the salt and pepper. Sauté for 2 to 3 minutes or until the okra begins to brown a little bit. Hit Cancel.

4. Add the garlic, oregano, tomatoes and their juices, and 1 cup of water to the pot. Stir, then close and lock the lid of the pressure cooker. Set the valve to sealing.

5. Cook on high pressure for 20 minutes.

6. When the cooking is complete, hit Cancel and quick release the pressure.

7. Once the pin drops, unlock and remove the lid.

8. Hit Sauté and add the sausage and shrimp to the pot. Cook, uncovered, for about 5 minutes or until the shrimp is opaque and the sausage is hot.

9. Sprinkle with the parsley and serve.

Make-ahead tip: Prepare the recipe through step 7. Let the stew cool, then refrigerate or freeze it. When you are ready to eat, reheat the stew on the stovetop. When it's hot, add the sausage and shrimp. Cook until the shrimp is opaque and the sausage is hot. Sprinkle with the parsley and serve.

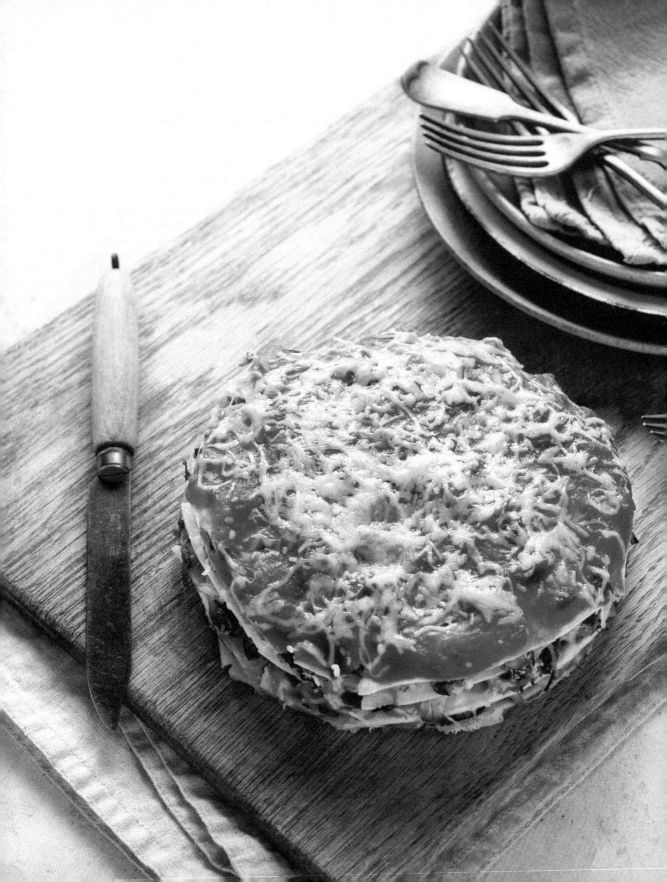

6

Meat

PREP TIME:
15 minutes

COOK SETTINGS:
Sauté, High

SAUTÉ TIME:
8 minutes

PRESSURE-UP TIME: 16 minutes

COOK TIME:
30 minutes

RELEASE: Natural for 10 minutes

TOTAL TIME:
1 hour 21 minutes

20-MINUTES-OR-LESS PREP

GLUTEN FREE

FAMILY FRIENDLY

**PER SERVING
(1½ CUPS):**
Calories: 268;
Total Fat: 10g; Protein: 25g;
Carbohydrates: 26g;
Sugars: 7g; Fiber: 7g;
Sodium: 387mg

Spicy Beef Stew with Butternut Squash

SERVES 8 (26G CARBS PER SERVING)

This is not your mother's beef stew. For one thing, there are no carrots or potatoes. For another, this version, featuring Moroccan spices, brings some heat. While the stew is perfect with beef, I've also found that pork tenderloin is equally delicious. The recipe makes a ton; freeze some for a quick meal on a busy day.

1½ tablespoons smoked paprika

2 teaspoons ground cinnamon

1½ teaspoons kosher salt

1 teaspoon ground ginger

1 teaspoon red pepper flakes

½ teaspoon freshly ground black pepper

2 pounds beef shoulder roast, cut into 1-inch cubes

2 tablespoons avocado oil, divided

1 cup low-sodium beef or vegetable broth

1 medium red onion, cut into wedges

8 garlic cloves, minced

1 (28-ounce) carton or can no-salt-added diced tomatoes

2 pounds butternut squash, peeled and cut into 1-inch pieces

Chopped fresh cilantro or parsley, for serving

1. In a zip-top bag or medium bowl, combine the paprika, cinnamon, salt, ginger, red pepper, and black pepper. Add the beef and toss to coat.

2. Set the electric pressure cooker to the Sauté setting. When the pot is hot, pour in 1 tablespoon of avocado oil.

3. Add half of the beef to the pot and cook, stirring occasionally, for 3 to 5 minutes or until the beef is no longer pink. Transfer it to a plate, then add the remaining 1 tablespoon of avocado oil and brown the remaining beef. Transfer to the plate. Hit Cancel.

4. Stir in the broth and scrape up any brown bits from the bottom of the pot. Return the beef to the pot and add the onion, garlic, tomatoes and their juices, and squash. Stir well.

5. Close and lock lid of pressure cooker. Set the valve to sealing.

6. Cook on high pressure for 30 minutes.

7. When cooking is complete, hit Cancel. Allow the pressure to release naturally for 10 minutes, then quick release any remaining pressure.

8. Unlock and remove lid.

9. Spoon into serving bowls, sprinkle with cilantro or parsley, and serve.

Make-ahead tip: Mix up your spices, peel and chop the squash, and cut the beef into cubes the night before. You could also look for prechopped squash (fresh or frozen) and precut beef (stew beef).

Mary's Meatloaf

SERVES 6 (21G CARBS PER SERVING)

This is the first of two beef dishes contributed by nutritionist and chef Mary Opfer, RD, CDN. It's not often that you find someone who is both a dietitian *and* a professionally trained chef, so I was thrilled when Mary offered her recipes. My husband, a true meatloaf fan, gives Mary's version a big thumbs-up. About the only thing I changed about this recipe was using my own Spiced Tomato Ketchup (page 123).

¼ cup breadcrumbs

⅓ cup 2% milk

2 large shallots, grated on the large holes of a box grater (about ¾ cup)

2 large eggs, lightly beaten

½ teaspoon salt

½ teaspoon freshly ground black pepper

1½ pounds ground chuck steak

8 ounces ground sirloin

¼ cup Spiced Tomato Ketchup (page 123) or ketchup

PREP TIME:
17 minutes

COOK SETTING:
High

PRESSURE-UP TIME: 8 minutes

COOK TIME:
35 minutes

RELEASE: Quick

TOTAL TIME:
1 hour 6 minutes

SPECIAL EQUIPMENT:
meat thermometer

20-MINUTES-OR-LESS PREP

FAMILY FRIENDLY

PER SERVING:
Calories: 340;
Total Fat: 15g; Protein: 29g;
Carbohydrates: 21g;
Sugars: 3g; Fiber: 1g;
Sodium: 371mg

1. In a large bowl, combine the breadcrumbs and milk. Let the mixture stand for 5 minutes. Meanwhile, tear off an 18-inch-long piece of foil, then fold it in half lengthwise to form an 18-by-6-inch rectangle. Grease the foil.

2. To the breadcrumb mixture, add the shallots, eggs, salt, and pepper. Stir to combine.

3. Add the ground chuck and ground sirloin. Mix with your hands until it holds together. (At first it might seem too wet; keep mixing until it comes together.)

4. Pour 2 cups of water into the electric pressure cooker and insert a wire rack or trivet.

5. Place the meat mixture in the center of the foil and shape it into a 7-by-5-inch loaf. Using the foil as a sling, lower the meatloaf into the pot onto the rack. Spread the ketchup on top of the meatloaf.

6. Close and lock the lid of the pressure cooker. Set the valve to sealing.

7. Cook on high pressure for 35 minutes.

8. When the cooking is complete, hit Cancel and quick release the pressure.

9. Once the pin drops, unlock and remove the lid.

10. Check the internal temperature of the meatloaf. If it is not at least 155°F, replace the lid and cook on high pressure for an additional 5 minutes.

11. Lift the meatloaf out of the pressure cooker onto a cutting board and let it rest for 5 minutes.

12. Slice and serve.

Ingredient tip: Mary recommends Aleia's gluten-free breadcrumbs for their coarse texture.

PREP TIME:
15 minutes

COOK SETTINGS:
Sauté, High

SAUTÉ TIME:
6 minutes

PRESSURE-UP TIME: 13 minutes

COOK TIME:
20 minutes

RELEASE: Natural for 10 minutes, then Quick

TOTAL TIME:
1 hour 10 minutes

20-MINUTES-OR-LESS PREP

FAMILY FRIENDLY

**PER SERVING
(1¼ CUPS):**
Calories: 321;
Total Fat: 13g; Protein: 11g;
Carbohydrates: 42g;
Sugars: 7g; Fiber: 11g;
Sodium: 412mg

Corned Beef and Cabbage Soup with Barley

SERVES 4 (42G CARBS PER SERVING)

Is corned beef, cabbage, and potatoes a favorite meal? You can still enjoy it—just think of the high-fat, high-sodium corned beef more as a garnish instead of the main event, swapping high-fiber barley for potatoes. If you don't happen to have any leftover corned beef lying around, visit the deli counter and ask for a quarter pound unsliced.

2 tablespoons avocado oil

1 small onion, chopped

3 celery stalks, chopped

3 medium carrots, chopped

¼ teaspoon allspice

4 cups Chicken Bone Broth (page 117), Vegetable Broth (page 116), low-sodium store-bought beef broth, or water

4 cups sliced green cabbage (about ⅓ medium head)

¾ cup pearled barley

4 ounces cooked corned beef, cut into thin strips or chunks

Freshly ground black pepper

1. Set the electric pressure cooker to the Sauté setting. When the pot is hot, pour in the avocado oil.

2. Sauté the onion, celery, and carrots for 3 to 5 minutes or until the vegetables begin to soften. Stir in the allspice. Hit Cancel.

3. Stir in the broth, cabbage, and barley.

4. Close and lock the lid of the pressure cooker. Set the valve to sealing.

5. Cook on high pressure for 20 minutes.

6. When the cooking is complete, allow the pressure to release naturally for 10 minutes, then quick release any remaining pressure. Hit Cancel.

7. Once the pin drops, unlock and remove the lid.

8. Stir in the corned beef, season with pepper, and replace the lid. Let the soup sit for about 5 minutes to let the corned beef warm up.

9. Spoon into serving bowls and serve.

Repurpose tip: If you're like me, you cook corned beef precisely once a year, usually sometime near St. Patrick's Day. The problem is always what to do with the leftovers. One solution is to make this soup.

Korean-Inspired Beef

SERVES 6 (13G CARBS PER SERVING)

When my brother was in the US Air Force, he spent some time in South Korea and came home talking about a spicy beef dish called *bulgogi*. Try serving this savory beef with fresh, crunchy vegetables like bean sprouts, shredded carrots, and spiralized zucchini.

¼ cup low-sodium beef broth or Vegetable Broth (page 116)

¼ cup low-sodium gluten-free tamari or soy sauce

2 tablespoons rice wine vinegar

2 teaspoons Sriracha sauce (optional)

2 tablespoons brown sugar

1 tablespoon sesame oil

3 tablespoons minced garlic

1 tablespoon peeled and minced fresh ginger

½ teaspoon onion powder

1 teaspoon freshly ground black pepper

2 pounds top round beef, cut into thin, 3-inch-long strips

2 tablespoons cornstarch

1 teaspoon sesame seeds

2 scallions, green parts only, thinly sliced

PREP TIME:
10 minutes

COOK SETTINGS:
High, Sauté

PRESSURE-UP TIME: 12 minutes

COOK TIME:
10 minutes

RELEASE: Quick

TOTAL TIME:
38 minutes

20-MINUTES-OR-LESS PREP

GLUTEN FREE

FAMILY FRIENDLY

PER SERVING:
Calories: 328;
Total Fat: 15g; Protein: 35g;
Carbohydrates: 13g;
Sugars: 4g; Fiber: 2g;
Sodium: 490mg

1. In a 2-cup measuring cup or medium bowl, whisk together the broth, tamari, vinegar, Sriracha (if using), brown sugar, sesame oil, garlic, ginger, onion powder, and pepper.

2. In the electric pressure cooker, combine the beef and broth mixture; stir.

3. Close and lock the lid of the pressure cooker. Set the valve to sealing.

4. Cook on high pressure for 10 minutes.

5. When the cooking is complete, hit Cancel and quick release the pressure.

6. Once the pin drops, unlock and remove the lid.

7. Using a slotted spoon, transfer the beef to a serving bowl. Hit Sauté/More.

8. In a small bowl, combine the cornstarch and 3 tablespoons of cold water to make a slurry. Whisk the cornstarch mixture into the liquid in the pot and cook, stirring frequently, for about 2 minutes or until the sauce has thickened. Hit Cancel.

9. Pour the sauce over the beef and garnish with the sesame seeds and scallions.

Ingredient tip: Look for presliced "Top Round for Stir-Fry" in the meat department of your grocery store to save yourself some prep time.

Mary's Sunday Pot Roast

SERVES 10 (6G CARBS PER SERVING)

PREP TIME:
10 minutes

COOK SETTINGS:
Sauté, High

SAUTÉ TIME:
15 minutes

PRESSURE-UP TIME: 15 minutes

COOK TIME:
1 hour 30 minutes

RELEASE: Natural

TOTAL TIME:
2 hours 49 minutes

20-MINUTES-OR-LESS PREP

LOW CARB

FAMILY FRIENDLY

PER SERVING:
Calories: 245;
Total Fat: 10g; Protein: 33g;
Carbohydrates: 6g;
Sugars: 2g; Fiber: 1g;
Sodium: 397mg

When you're craving good old-fashioned pot roast, try this version from nutritionist and chef Mary Opfer, RD, CDN (maryopfernutrition.com). Even though there are only two of us in the house, I like to cook a 4-pound roast for Sunday dinner and use the leftover beef in other dishes throughout the week. Nothing beats a cook-once-eat-several-meals recipe.

1 (3- to 4-pound) beef rump roast

2 teaspoons kosher salt, divided

2 tablespoons avocado oil

1 large onion, coarsely chopped (about 1½ cups)

4 large carrots, each cut into 4 pieces

1 tablespoon minced garlic

3 cups low-sodium beef broth

1 teaspoon freshly ground black pepper

1 tablespoon dried parsley

2 tablespoons all-purpose flour

1. Rub the roast all over with 1 teaspoon of the salt.

2. Set the electric pressure cooker to the Sauté setting. When the pot is hot, pour in the avocado oil.

3. Carefully place the roast in the pot and sear it for 6 to 9 minutes on each side. (You want a dark caramelized crust.) Hit Cancel.

4. Transfer the roast from the pot to a plate.

5. In order, put the onion, carrots, and garlic in the pot. Place the roast on top of the vegetables along with any juices that accumulated on the plate.

6. In a medium bowl, whisk together the broth, remaining 1 teaspoon of salt, pepper, and parsley. Pour the broth mixture over the roast.

7. Close and lock the lid of the pressure cooker. Set the valve to sealing.

8. Cook on high pressure for 1 hour and 30 minutes.

9. When the cooking is complete, hit Cancel and allow the pressure to release naturally.

10. Once the pin drops, unlock and remove the lid.

11. Using large slotted spoons, transfer the roast and vegetables to a serving platter while you make the gravy.

12. Using a large spoon or fat separator, remove the fat from the juices in the pot. Set the electric pressure cooker to the Sauté setting and bring the liquid to a boil.

13. In a small bowl, whisk together the flour and 4 tablespoons of water to make a slurry. Pour the slurry into the pot, whisking occasionally, until the gravy is the thickness you like. Season with salt and pepper, if necessary.

14. Serve the meat and carrots with the gravy.

Repurpose tip: Try some of the leftover shredded beef in 5-Ingredient Mexican Lasagna (page 101), lettuce or cabbage wraps, and tacos.

PREP TIME:
10 minutes

COOK SETTINGS:
Sauté, High

SAUTÉ TIME:
9 minutes

**PRESSURE-UP
TIME:** 6 minutes

COOK TIME:
20 minutes

RELEASE: Natural
for 15 minutes,
then Quick

TOTAL TIME:
1 hour

**20-MINUTES-OR-
LESS PREP**

GLUTEN FREE

LOW CARB

FAMILY FRIENDLY

PER SERVING:
Calories: 150;
Total Fat: 5g; Protein: 22g;
Carbohydrates: 3g;
Sugars: 1g; Fiber: 1g;
Sodium: 245mg

Pork Carnitas

SERVES 8 (3G CARBS PER SERVING)

Pork butt (Boston butt), a fatty cut from the upper shoulder of a pig, is typically used to make pulled pork and carnitas, a Mexican style of pulled pork usually braised in oil. If you want to save yourself some saturated fat, look for a leaner pork sirloin roast instead, which comes from the top of the pig (toward the rear). If you decide to go with butt, get a boneless one—having to cut around a bone will add significantly to your prep time.

1 teaspoon kosher salt

2 teaspoons chili powder

2 teaspoons dried oregano

½ teaspoon freshly ground
black pepper

1 (2½-pound) pork sirloin roast
or boneless pork butt, cut into
1½-inch cubes

2 tablespoons avocado oil, divided

3 garlic cloves, minced

Juice and zest of 1 large orange

Juice and zest of 1 medium lime

6-inch gluten-free corn tortillas,
warmed, for serving (optional)

Chopped avocado, for serving
(optional)

Roasted Tomatillo Salsa (page 121) or
salsa verde, for serving (optional)

Shredded cheddar cheese, for serving
(optional)

1. In a large bowl or gallon-size zip-top bag, combine the salt, chili powder, oregano, and pepper. Add the pork cubes and toss to coat.

2. Set the electric pressure cooker to the Sauté/More setting. When the pot is hot, pour in 1 tablespoon of avocado oil.

3. Add half of the pork to the pot and sear until the pork is browned on all sides, about 5 minutes. Transfer the pork to a plate, add the remaining 1 tablespoon of avocado oil to the pot, and sear the remaining pork. Hit Cancel.

4. Return all of the pork to the pot and add the garlic, orange zest and juice, and lime zest and juice to the pot.

5. Close and lock the lid of the pressure cooker. Set the valve to sealing.

6. Cook on high pressure for 20 minutes.

7. When the cooking is complete, hit Cancel. Allow the pressure to release naturally for 15 minutes then quick release any remaining pressure.

8. Once the pin drops, unlock and remove the lid.

9. Using two forks, shred the meat right in the pot.

10. (Optional) For more authentic carnitas, spread the shredded meat on a broiler-safe sheet pan. Preheat the broiler with the rack 6 inches from the heating element. Broil the pork for about 5 minutes or until it begins to crisp. (Watch carefully so you don't let the pork burn.)

11. Place the pork in a serving bowl. Top with some of the juices from the pot. Serve with tortillas, avocado, salsa, and cheddar cheese (if using).

Repurpose tip: Use leftovers in the 4-Ingredient Carnitas Posole (page 45).

Sweet and Sour Pork Chops

SERVES 4 (16G CARBS PER SERVING)

PREP TIME:
7 minutes

COOK SETTINGS:
Sauté, High

SAUTÉ TIME:
9 minutes

PRESSURE-UP TIME: 6 minutes

COOK TIME:
1 minute

RELEASE: Natural for 10 minutes, then Quick

TOTAL TIME:
43 minutes

SPECIAL EQUIPMENT:
meat tenderizing mallet, 2-cup liquid measuring cup

20-MINUTES-OR-LESS PREP

FAMILY FRIENDLY

PER SERVING:
Calories: 407;
Total Fat: 17g; Protein: 45g;
Carbohydrates: 16g;
Sugars: 11g; Fiber: 1g;
Sodium: 416mg

When I was first learning to cook, I made an easy version of sweet and sour pork using canned pineapple and Heinz 57 steak sauce. Here, I've tried to recreate a similar taste with a homemade sauce. I recommend mixing up the sauce ahead of time if you can to let the flavors blend. Make sure your pineapple is packed in juice, not heavy syrup.

For the sauce

3 tablespoons Spiced Tomato Ketchup (page 123) or store-bought ketchup

1 tablespoon Worcestershire sauce

1 teaspoon yellow mustard

½ teaspoon freshly squeezed lemon juice

Few drops hot pepper sauce (optional)

For the pork chops

4 (¾-inch-thick) rib pork chops

Kosher salt

Freshly ground black pepper

2 tablespoons avocado oil, divided

1 (8-ounce) can pineapple chunks in juice

2 tablespoons cornstarch

1 medium green bell pepper, cut into thin strips

To make the sauce

In a 2-cup liquid measuring cup or small bowl, mix together the ketchup, Worcestershire sauce, mustard, lemon juice, and hot pepper sauce (if using).

To make the pork chops

1. Set the electric pressure cooker to the Sauté setting. Sprinkle both sides of pork chops with salt and pepper and use a meat tenderizing mallet to pound both sides. (If you don't have a mallet, you can use a rolling pin, or try my grandpa's trick of using the edge of a small plate.) When the pot is hot, pour in 1 tablespoon of avocado oil.

2. Add 2 pork chops to the pot in a single layer and brown for 2 to 3 minutes per side. Transfer the pork chops to a plate. Repeat with the remaining avocado oil and pork chops. Hit Cancel.

3. Drain the pineapple juice from the can into a 2-cup liquid measuring cup. Add enough water so that you have 1 cup of liquid. Pour this into the pot and scrape up any browned bits that are stuck to the bottom. Set the pineapple chunks aside.

4. Return the pork chops to the pot (overlapping them is fine); pour some of the sauce mixture on top of each one.

5. Close and lock the lid of the pressure cooker. Set the valve to sealing.

6. Cook on high pressure for 1 minute.

7. When the cooking is complete, allow the pressure to release naturally for 10 minutes, then quick release any remaining pressure. Hit Cancel.

8. Once the pin drops, unlock and remove the lid.

9. Remove the pork chops from the pot. Hit Sauté.

10. In a small bowl, mix together the cornstarch and 3 tablespoons of cold water to make a slurry. Add it to the pot and cook, stirring frequently, for a few minutes, until the mixture begins to thicken.

11. Add the reserved pineapple and green pepper to the pot. Cook, stirring occasionally, for about 5 minutes or until the green pepper softens. Hit Cancel. Return the pork chops to the pot and coat with sauce.

12. Place the pork chops on serving plates, top with sauce, and serve.

Substitution tip: You can use ⅓ cup Heinz 57 steak sauce instead of the homemade sauce, but this will add a lot more sodium to the dish.

Balsamic Pork Tenderloin with Raisins

SERVES 4 (13G CARBS PER SERVING)

I thought trying to cook pork tenderloin in an EPC was hopeless until I learned the secret from Amy and Jacky of PressureCookRecipes.com. Just use a cook time of 0 minutes with a natural Pressure release of 15 minutes, then let the meat rest for 10 minutes before slicing. The result will be some of the juiciest pork tenderloin you've ever eaten. Do not skip the resting phase or your pork will be tough. Trust me.

PREP TIME:
8 minutes

COOK SETTINGS:
Sauté, High

SAUTÉ TIME:
8 minutes

PRESSURE-UP TIME: 5 minutes

COOK TIME:
0 minutes

RELEASE: Natural for 15 minutes, then Quick

TOTAL TIME:
36 minutes

SPECIAL EQUIPMENT:
meat thermometer

20-MINUTES-OR-LESS PREP

GLUTEN FREE

FAMILY FRIENDLY

PER SERVING:
Calories: 300;
Total Fat: 11g; Protein: 36g;
Carbohydrates: 13g;
Sugars: 10g; Fiber: 1g;
Sodium: 186mg

1½ pounds pork tenderloin (1 tenderloin)

Kosher salt

Freshly ground black pepper

2 tablespoons avocado oil

½ cup unsweetened apple juice or apple cider

1 teaspoon herbes de Provence

½ teaspoon garlic powder

1 tablespoon balsamic vinegar

¼ cup unsweetened applesauce or Spiced Pear Applesauce (page 105)

¼ cup golden raisins

1. Trim the silver skin from the side of the tenderloin, if necessary. Cut the tenderloin in half crosswise. Season both pieces all over with salt and pepper.

2. Set the electric pressure cooker to the Sauté/More setting. When the pot is hot, pour in the avocado oil.

3. Add the tenderloin pieces to the pot and brown for 5 minutes without turning. Flip and brown the other sides for about 3 minutes. Hit Cancel. Transfer the pork to a plate.

4. Add the apple juice to the pot and scrape up any brown bits from the bottom.

5. Stir in the herbes de Provence, garlic powder, vinegar, applesauce, and raisins. Return the pork to the pot and nestle it into the liquid.

6. Close and lock the lid of the pressure cooker. Set the valve to sealing.

7. Cook on high pressure for 0 minutes (the additional cooking will all occur as the pressure cooker comes to pressure and then naturally releases).

8. When the cooking is complete, hit Cancel. Allow the pressure to release naturally for 15 minutes, then quick release any remaining pressure.

9. Once the pin drops, unlock and remove the lid. Use a meat thermometer to check the internal temperature of the pork. If the pork's temperature is at least 137°F, flip the pork over, replace the lid and let the meat rest for 10 minutes. (The temperature should continue to rise to a safe serving temperature of 145°F.) If the pork's temperature is less than 137°F, hit Sauté to turn the pressure cooker back on. Cook the pork, turning occasionally, until it reaches a temperature of 137°F. Hit Cancel. Replace the lid and let the meat rest for 10 minutes.

10. Transfer the pork to a cutting board. Thinly slice and serve topped with raisins and sauce.

Substitution tip: No apple juice or apple cider handy? Use low-sodium chicken broth, vegetable broth, or water. You do have some Chicken Bone Broth (page 117) or Vegetable Broth (page 116) in your freezer, right?

Rosemary Lamb Chops

SERVES 4 (1G CARBS PER SERVING)

PREP TIME:
25 minutes

COOK SETTINGS:
Sauté, High

SAUTÉ TIME:
9 minutes

**PRESSURE-UP
TIME:** 6 minutes

COOK TIME:
2 minutes

RELEASE: Quick

TOTAL TIME:
44 minutes

GLUTEN FREE

LOW CARB

FAMILY FRIENDLY

**PER SERVING
(1 LAMB CHOP):**
Calories: 233;
Total Fat: 18g;
Protein: 15g;
Carbohydrates: 1g;
Sugars: 1; Fiber: 0g;
Sodium: 450mg

I'm not a huge lamb fan, but during one shopping trip, I saw some cute little chops at the store and decided to surprise my husband. He's big into rosemary, so I got double points when I made him this dish for dinner. Look for tomato paste in a tube or 2-tablespoon pouches—both are handy when you don't need an entire 6-ounce can.

1½ pounds lamb chops (4 small chops)

1 teaspoon kosher salt

Leaves from 1 (6-inch) rosemary sprig

2 tablespoons avocado oil

1 shallot, peeled and cut in quarters

1 tablespoon tomato paste

1 cup beef broth

1. Place the lamb chops on a cutting board. Press the salt and rosemary leaves into both sides of the chops. Let rest at room temperature for 15 to 30 minutes.
2. Set the electric pressure cooker to Sauté/More setting. When hot, add the avocado oil.
3. Brown the lamb chops, about 2 minutes per side. (If they don't all fit in a single layer, brown them in batches.)
4. Transfer the chops to a plate. In the pot, combine the shallot, tomato paste, and broth. Cook for about a minute, scraping up the brown bits from the bottom. Hit Cancel.
5. Add the chops and any accumulated juices back to the pot.
6. Close and lock the lid of the pressure cooker. Set the valve to sealing.
7. Cook on high pressure for 2 minutes.
8. When the cooking is complete, hit Cancel and quick release the pressure.
9. Once the pin drops, unlock and remove the lid.
10. Place the lamb chops on plates and serve immediately.

Substitution tip: No shallots? Use a few thin slices of onion instead.

5-Ingredient Mexican Lasagna

SERVES 4 (34G CARBS PER SERVING)

In this "lasagna," gluten-free corn tortillas replace the noodles and salsa pinch hits for the pasta sauce. It's a great way to use up leftover meat, or you can try a whole can of beans and skip the meat entirely for a vegetarian option. Your salsa can be mild, medium, or hot, depending on your preference. If you like things spicy, try pepper Jack cheese.

Nonstick cooking spray

½ (15-ounce) can light red kidney beans, rinsed and drained

4 (6-inch) gluten-free corn tortillas

1½ cups cooked shredded beef, pork, or chicken

1⅓ cups salsa

1⅓ cups shredded Mexican cheese blend

PREP TIME:
15 minutes

COOK SETTING:
High

PRESSURE-UP TIME: 6 minutes

COOK TIME:
15 minutes

RELEASE: Natural for 10 minutes, then Quick

TOTAL TIME:
51 minutes

SPECIAL EQUIPMENT:
6-inch springform pan

20-MINUTES-OR-LESS PREP

GLUTEN FREE

FAMILY FRIENDLY

PER SERVING:
Calories: 395;
Total Fat: 16g; Protein: 30g;
Carbohydrates: 34g;
Sugars: 5g; Fiber: 9g;
Sodium: 1140mg

1. Spray a 6-inch springform pan with nonstick spray. Wrap the bottom in foil.

2. In a medium bowl, mash the beans with a fork.

3. Place 1 tortilla in the bottom of the pan. Add about ⅓ of the beans, ½ cup of meat, ⅓ cup of salsa, and ⅓ cup of cheese. Press down. Repeat for 2 more layers. Add the remaining tortilla and press down. Top with the remaining salsa and cheese. There are no beans or meat on the top layer.

4. Tear off a piece of foil big enough to cover the pan, and spray it with nonstick spray. Line the pan with the foil, sprayed-side down.

5. Pour 1 cup of water into the electric pressure cooker.

6. Place the pan on the wire rack and carefully lower it into the pot. Close and lock the lid of the pressure cooker. Set the valve to sealing.

7. Cook on high pressure for 15 minutes.

8. When the cooking is complete, hit Cancel. Allow the pressure to release naturally for 10 minutes, then quick release any remaining pressure.

9. Once the pin drops, unlock and remove the lid.

10. Using the handles of the wire rack, carefully remove the pan from the pot. Let the lasagna sit for 5 minutes. Carefully remove the ring.

11. Slice into quarters and serve.

Repurpose tip: Use any shredded beef, pork, or chicken in this recipe. Try leftovers from Mary's Sunday Pot Roast (page 92), Pork Carnitas (page 94), or Smoky Whole Chicken (page 70).

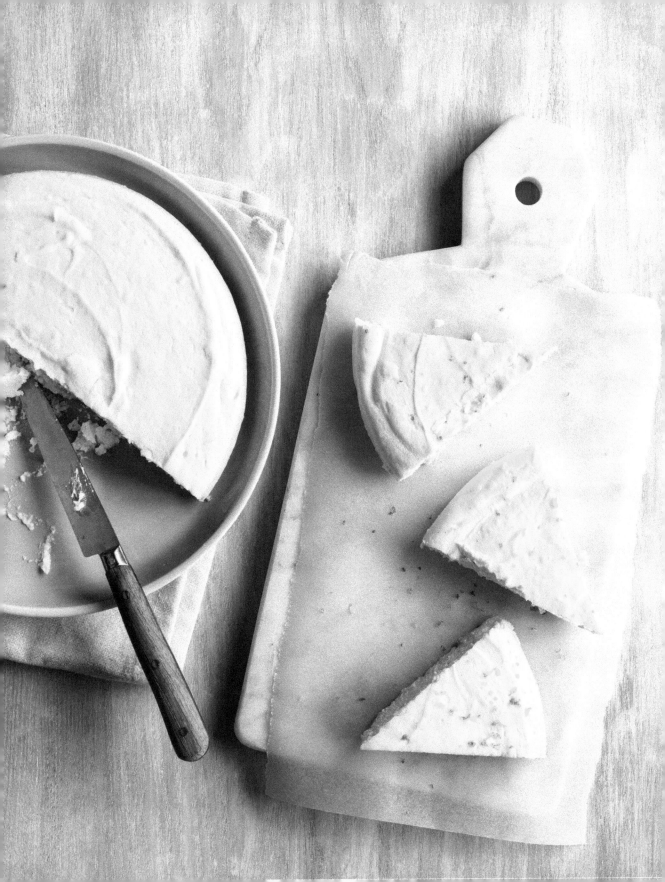

7

Desserts

Apple Crunch

SERVES 4 (26G CARBS PER SERVING)

PREP TIME:
13 minutes

COOK SETTING:
High

**PRESSURE-UP
TIME:** 7 minutes

COOK TIME:
2 minutes

RELEASE: Quick

TOTAL TIME:
24 minutes

**20-MINUTES-OR-
LESS PREP**

VEGAN

FAMILY FRIENDLY

LOW SODIUM

PER SERVING:
Calories: 103;
Total Fat: 1g; Protein: 1g;
Carbohydrates: 26g;
Sugars: 18g; Fiber: 4g;
Sodium: 13mg

The fruits I eat most often are apples, pears, and berries, although I do indulge in fresh peaches and nectarines when they are in season. This simple dessert could easily be made with any summer stone fruit. As with all sweets, watch your portion size.

3 apples, peeled, cored, and sliced (about 1½ pounds)

1 teaspoon pure maple syrup

1 teaspoon apple pie spice or ground cinnamon

¼ cup unsweetened apple juice, apple cider, or water

¼ cup low-sugar granola

1. In the electric pressure cooker, combine the apples, maple syrup, apple pie spice, and apple juice.
2. Close and lock the lid of the pressure cooker. Set the valve to sealing.
3. Cook on high pressure for 2 minutes.
4. When the cooking is complete, hit Cancel and quick release the pressure.
5. Once the pin drops, unlock and remove the lid.
6. Spoon the apples into 4 serving bowls and sprinkle each with 1 tablespoon of granola.

Ingredient tip: Granola is one of those foods that sounds really healthy but is usually loaded with sugar. Look for a brand that's high in fiber and low in sugar, or make your own. You can also top your apples with nuts and seeds or crumbled breakfast cereal (low-carb, of course!) instead of granola.

Spiced Pear Applesauce

MAKES 3½ CUPS (29G CARBS PER SERVING)

Who needs applesauce from a jar when making your own is so easy? It's also a good way to guarantee that there's no added sugar. You can use this recipe to make pear applesauce, regular applesauce, or pear sauce. You could throw in some peaches or mango, too. Just make sure to use 3 pounds of fruit total.

2 pounds apples, peeled, cored, and sliced

1 pound pears, peeled, cored, and sliced

2 teaspoons apple pie spice or cinnamon

Pinch kosher salt

Juice of ½ small lemon

1. In the electric pressure cooker, combine the apples, pears, apple pie spice, salt, lemon juice, and ¼ cup of water.
2. Close and lock the lid of the pressure cooker. Set the valve to sealing.
3. Cook on high pressure for 5 minutes.
4. When the cooking is complete, hit Cancel and let the pressure release naturally.
5. Once the pin drops, unlock and remove the lid.
6. Mash the apples and pears with a potato masher to the consistency you like.
7. Serve warm, or cool to room temperature and refrigerate.

Repurpose tip: Try using your own homemade pear applesauce in Sweet and Sour Red Cabbage (page 32) or Balsamic Pork Tenderloin with Raisins (page 98). It's also great mixed into plain yogurt.

PREP TIME: 15 minutes

COOK SETTING: High

PRESSURE-UP TIME: 11 minutes

COOK TIME: 5 minutes

RELEASE: Natural

TOTAL TIME: 48 minutes

SPECIAL EQUIPMENT: potato masher

20-MINUTES-OR-LESS PREP

GLUTEN FREE

VEGAN

FAMILY FRIENDLY

LOW SODIUM

PER SERVING (½ CUP): Calories: 108; Total Fat: 1g; Protein: 1g; Carbohydrates: 29g; Sugars: 20g; Fiber: 6g; Sodium: 15mg

Chai Pear-Fig Compote

SERVES 4 (44G CARBS PER SERVING)

PREP TIME:
20 minutes

COOK SETTINGS:
Sauté, High

**PRESSURE-UP
TIME:** 7 minutes

COOK TIME:
3 minutes

RELEASE: Quick

TOTAL TIME:
31 minutes

20-MINUTES-OR-LESS PREP

GLUTEN FREE

VEGAN

FAMILY FRIENDLY

LOW SODIUM

PER SERVING:
Calories: 167;
Total Fat: 1g; Protein: 2g;
Carbohydrates: 44g;
Sugars: 29g; Fiber: 9g;
Sodium: 4mg

Before I met my husband, the only figs I'd ever had were dried. Then he introduced me to the fresh figs he picked from his neighbor's tree (with permission, of course), and a whole new world opened up. We even have a couple of fig trees of our own now. While figs do contain a lot of natural sugar, they are also loaded with nutrients (like vitamin B$_6$) and fiber.

1 vanilla chai tea bag

1 (3-inch) cinnamon stick

1 strip lemon peel (about 2-by-½ inches)

1½ pounds pears, peeled and chopped (about 3 cups)

½ cup chopped dried figs

2 tablespoons raisins

1. Pour 1 cup of water into the electric pressure cooker and hit Sauté/More. When the water comes to a boil, add the tea bag and cinnamon stick. Hit Cancel. Let the tea steep for 5 minutes, then remove and discard the tea bag.

2. Add the lemon peel, pears, figs, and raisins to the pot.

3. Close and lock the lid of the pressure cooker. Set the valve to sealing.

4. Cook on high pressure for 3 minutes.

5. When the cooking is complete, hit Cancel and quick release the pressure.

6. Once the pin drops, unlock and remove the lid.

7. Remove the lemon peel and cinnamon stick. Serve warm or cool to room temperature and refrigerate.

Ingredient tip: Believe it or not, there are more than 150 varieties of figs in the world. The most common are Black Mission (deep purple skin and pink flesh) and Brown Turkey (purplish-brown skin and red flesh). Any dried figs will work in this recipe, but make sure to cut off the stems.

Goat Cheese–Stuffed Pears

SERVES 4 (17G CARBS PER SERVING)

The easiest way I've found to core a pear is to use a melon baller; just cut the pear in half lengthwise and then scoop out the seedy area. The resulting space is the perfect spot for a dollop of goat cheese. If you don't have any pistachios, try walnuts or almonds instead. This dessert is the perfect blend of creamy, sweet, and crunchy.

2 ounces goat cheese, at room temperature

2 teaspoons pure maple syrup

2 ripe, firm pears, halved lengthwise and cored

2 tablespoons chopped pistachios, toasted (see page 120)

1. Pour 1 cup of water into the electric pressure cooker and insert a wire rack or trivet.
2. In a small bowl, combine the goat cheese and maple syrup.
3. Spoon the goat cheese mixture into the cored pear halves. Place the pears on the rack inside the pot, cut-side up.
4. Close and lock the lid of the pressure cooker. Set the valve to sealing.
5. Cook on high pressure for 2 minutes.
6. When the cooking is complete, hit Cancel and quick release the pressure.
7. Once the pin drops, unlock and remove the lid.
8. Using tongs, carefully transfer the pears to serving plates.
9. Sprinkle with pistachios and serve immediately.

Ingredient tip: My favorite pears to use in this recipe are Boscs, but I often have a hard time finding them unbruised. I've also used Anjou (both red and green) with success. Pick pears that are ripe but still firm.

PREP TIME:
6 minutes

COOK SETTING:
High

PRESSURE-UP TIME: 9 minutes

COOK TIME:
2 minutes

RELEASE: Quick

TOTAL TIME:
18 minutes

20-MINUTES-OR-LESS PREP

GLUTEN FREE

FAMILY FRIENDLY

LOW SODIUM

PER SERVING
(½ **PEAR**): Calories: 120; Total Fat: 5g; Protein: 4g; Carbohydrates: 17g; Sugars: 11g; Fiber: 3g; Sodium: 54mg

PREP TIME:
10 minutes

COOK SETTING:
High

PRESSURE-UP TIME: 7 minutes

COOK TIME:
6 minutes

RELEASE: Natural for 10 minutes, then Quick

TOTAL TIME:
33 minutes, plus 2 hours chilling

20-MINUTES-OR-LESS PREP

GLUTEN FREE

VEGAN

FAMILY FRIENDLY

LOW SODIUM

**PER SERVING
(6 TABLESPOONS
TAPIOCA,
½ CUP BERRIES,
AND 1 TABLESPOON
ALMONDS):**
Calories: 174;
Total Fat: 5g; Protein: 3g;
Carbohydrates: 32g;
Sugars: 11g; Fiber: 3g;
Sodium: 77mg

Tapioca Berry Parfaits

SERVES 4 (32G CARBS PER SERVING)

The hardest part of making these parfaits is finding the small pearl tapioca. Fresh Market came through for me after I struck out at two other stores. You might want to order it online and save yourself some driving. Use your favorite berries or a combination. I like blueberries and sliced strawberries, especially when they're in season. Frozen berries will work, but thaw them first.

2 cups unsweetened almond milk

½ cup small pearl tapioca, rinsed and still wet

1 teaspoon almond extract

1 tablespoon pure maple syrup

2 cups berries

¼ cup slivered almonds

1. Pour the almond milk into the electric pressure cooker. Stir in the tapioca and almond extract.

2. Close and lock the lid of the pressure cooker. Set the valve to sealing.

3. Cook on High pressure for 6 minutes.

4. When the cooking is complete, hit Cancel. Allow the pressure to release naturally for 10 minutes, then quick release any remaining pressure.

5. Once the pin drops, unlock and remove the lid. Remove the pot to a cooling rack.

6. Stir in the maple syrup and let the mixture cool for about an hour.

7. In small glasses, create several layers of tapioca, berries, and almonds. Refrigerate for 1 hour.

8. Serve chilled.

Ingredient tip: Tapioca is made by extracting starch from the yuca root (cassava). It comes in four primary forms: large pearls, small pearls, instant, and flour. The large pearls are seen most often in bubble tea. The small pearls are featured in tapioca pudding. The instant variety and the flour (which is gluten-free) can be used as thickeners.

Chocolate Chip Banana Cake

SERVES 8 (39G CARBS PER SERVING)

Is this a cake or a bread? It has the texture of banana bread, but it's round, so I'm going with cake. If you plan to have this cake as dessert after a meal, make sure your meal is extremely low carb. Did you buy a bunch of bananas and not use them all before they started to turn dark in spots? Peel and freeze them. They won't look pretty, but they will work perfectly well in this cake or in smoothies.

Nonstick cooking spray

3 ripe bananas

½ cup buttermilk

3 tablespoons honey

1 teaspoon vanilla extract

2 large eggs, lightly beaten

3 tablespoons extra-virgin olive oil

1½ cups whole wheat pastry flour

⅛ teaspoon ground nutmeg

1 teaspoon ground cinnamon

¼ teaspoon salt

1 teaspoon baking soda

⅓ cup dark chocolate chips

1. Spray a 7-inch Bundt pan with nonstick cooking spray.
2. In a large bowl, mash the bananas. Add the buttermilk, honey, vanilla, eggs, and olive oil, and mix well.
3. In a medium bowl, whisk together the flour, nutmeg, cinnamon, salt, and baking soda.
4. Add the flour mixture to the banana mixture and mix well. Stir in the chocolate chips. Pour the batter into the prepared Bundt pan. Cover the pan with foil.
5. Pour 1 cup of water into the electric pressure cooker. Place the pan on the wire rack and lower it into the pressure cooker.
6. Close and lock the lid of the pressure cooker. Set the valve to sealing.
7. Cook on high pressure for 25 minutes.
8. When the cooking is complete, hit Cancel and quick release the pressure.
9. Once the pin drops, unlock and remove the lid.
10. Carefully transfer the pan to a cooling rack, uncover, and let it cool for 10 minutes.
11. Invert the cake onto the rack and let it cool for about an hour.
12. Slice and serve the cake.

Substitution tip: No buttermilk? Add ½ tablespoon of white vinegar to ½ cup of milk and let it sit for about 5 minutes.

PREP TIME:
15 minutes

COOK SETTING:
High

PRESSURE-UP TIME: 7 minutes

COOK TIME:
25 minutes

RELEASE: Quick

TOTAL TIME:
48 minutes, plus 1 hour cooling

SPECIAL EQUIPMENT:
7-inch Bundt pan

20-MINUTES-OR-LESS PREP

FAMILY FRIENDLY

**PER SERVING
(1 SLICE):** Calories: 261; Total Fat: 11g; Protein: 6g; Carbohydrates: 39g; Sugars: 16g; Fiber: 4g; Sodium: 239mg

Crustless Key Lime Cheesecake

SERVES 8 (4G CARBS PER SERVING)

PREP TIME:
15 minutes

COOK SETTING:
High

**PRESSURE-UP
TIME:** 6 minutes

COOK TIME:
35 minutes

RELEASE: Natural
for 20 minutes,
then Quick

TOTAL TIME:
1 hour 16 minutes,
plus 4 hours chilling

**SPECIAL
EQUIPMENT:**
7-inch
springform pan

20-MINUTES-OR-
LESS PREP

GLUTEN FREE

LOW CARB

FAMILY FRIENDLY

**PER SERVING
(1 SLICE):**
Calories: 157;
Total Fat: 12g; Protein: 8g;
Carbohydrates: 4g;
Sugars: 1g; Fiber: 0g;
Sodium: 196mg

Key lime pie is one of my favorite desserts. While the EPC isn't an ideal environment for pie, it is perfect for making cheesecake. You automatically get the steam that keeps baked cheesecakes from cracking without the hassle of concocting a water bath. I went crustless with this cheesecake to save myself some carbs. Did you know that the easiest way to slice a cheesecake is with dental floss? Try it.

Nonstick cooking spray

16 ounces light cream cheese (Neufchâtel), softened

⅔ cup granulated erythritol sweetener

¼ cup unsweetened Key lime juice (I like Nellie & Joe's Famous Key West Lime Juice)

½ teaspoon vanilla extract

¼ cup plain Greek yogurt

1 teaspoon grated lime zest

2 large eggs

Whipped cream, for garnish (optional)

1. Spray a 7-inch springform pan with nonstick cooking spray. Line the bottom and partway up the sides of the pan with foil.

2. Put the cream cheese in a large bowl. Use an electric mixer to whip the cream cheese until smooth, about 2 minutes. Add the erythritol, lime juice, vanilla, yogurt, and zest, and blend until smooth. Stop the mixer and scrape down the sides of the bowl with a rubber spatula. With the mixer on low speed, add the eggs, one at a time, blending until just mixed. (Don't overbeat the eggs.)

3. Pour the mixture into the prepared pan. Drape a paper towel over the top of the pan, not touching the cream cheese mixture, and tightly wrap the top of the pan in foil. (Your goal here is to keep out as much moisture as possible.)

4. Pour 1 cup of water into the electric pressure cooker.

5. Place the foil-covered pan onto the wire rack and carefully lower it into the pot.

6. Close and lock the lid of the pressure cooker. Set the valve to sealing.

7. Cook on high pressure for 35 minutes.

8. When the cooking is complete, hit Cancel. Allow the pressure to release naturally for 20 minutes, then quick release any remaining pressure.

9. Once the pin drops, unlock and remove the lid.

10. Using the handles of the wire rack, carefully transfer the pan to a cooling rack. Cool to room temperature, then refrigerate for at least 3 hours.

11. When ready to serve, run a thin rubber spatula around the rim of the cheese-cake to loosen it, then remove the ring.

12. Slice into wedges and serve with whipped cream (if using).

Ingredient tip: Erythritol is a sugar substitute in the sugar alcohol family. Low-carb bakers love it because it measures tablespoon-for-tablespoon like regular sugar (no conversions required). Most sugar substitutes I've tried wreak havoc on my digestive system, so I tend to avoid them. This is my first dive into the world of erythritol, which comes in granulated, powdered, and brown varieties. Look for it in health food stores, or online under the brand name Swerve™.

Chipotle Black Bean Brownies

SERVES 8 (29G CARBS PER SERVING)

PREP TIME:
15 minutes

COOK SETTING:
High

**PRESSURE-UP
TIME:** 7 minutes

COOK TIME:
30 minutes

RELEASE: Quick

TOTAL TIME:
53 minutes, plus
1 hour cooling

**SPECIAL
EQUIPMENT:**
7-inch Bundt pan

**20-MINUTES-OR-
LESS PREP**

FAMILY FRIENDLY

PER SERVING
(1 SLICE): Calories: 296;
Total Fat: 20g; Protein: 5g;
Carbohydrates: 29g;
Sugars: 16g; Fiber: 4g;
Sodium: 224mg

Here, you get the denseness of a brownie in the shape of a cake with an unexpected boost of fiber from the beans. If you like Mexican chocolate-chile bars, you'll love this dessert. The texture is a bit different from regular brownies (more spongy), and the flavor is very chocolatey but not too sweet.

Nonstick cooking spray

½ cup dark chocolate chips, divided

¾ cup cooked calypso beans or
    black beans

½ cup extra-virgin olive oil

2 large eggs

¼ cup unsweetened dark chocolate
    cocoa powder

⅓ cup honey

1 teaspoon vanilla extract

⅓ cup white wheat flour

½ teaspoon chipotle chili powder

½ teaspoon ground cinnamon

½ teaspoon baking powder

½ teaspoon kosher salt

1. Spray a 7-inch Bundt pan with nonstick cooking spray.

2. Place half of the chocolate chips in a small bowl and microwave them for 30 seconds. Stir and repeat, if necessary, until the chips have completely melted.

3. In a food processor, blend the beans and oil together. Add the melted chocolate chips, eggs, cocoa powder, honey, and vanilla. Blend until the mixture is smooth.

4. In a large bowl, whisk together the flour, chili powder, cinnamon, baking powder, and salt. Pour the bean mixture from the food processor into the bowl and stir with a wooden spoon until well combined. Stir in the remaining chocolate chips.

5. Pour the batter into the prepared Bundt pan. Cover loosely with foil.

6. Pour 1 cup of water into the electric pressure cooker.

7. Place the Bundt pan onto the wire rack and lower it into the pressure cooker.

8. Close and lock the lid of the pressure cooker. Set the valve to sealing.

9. Cook on high pressure for 30 minutes.

10. When the cooking is complete, hit Cancel and quick release the pressure.

11. Once the pin drops, unlock and remove the lid.

12. Carefully transfer the pan to a cooling rack for about 10 minutes, then invert the cake onto the rack and let it cool completely.

13. Cut into slices and serve.

Ingredient tip: I really like using black-and-white speckled calypso (orca) beans in this recipe, but they can be hard to find. If you're lucky enough to snag a bag, cook them according to the guidelines for black beans in Salt-Free No-Soak Beans (page 64). Otherwise, just use black beans.

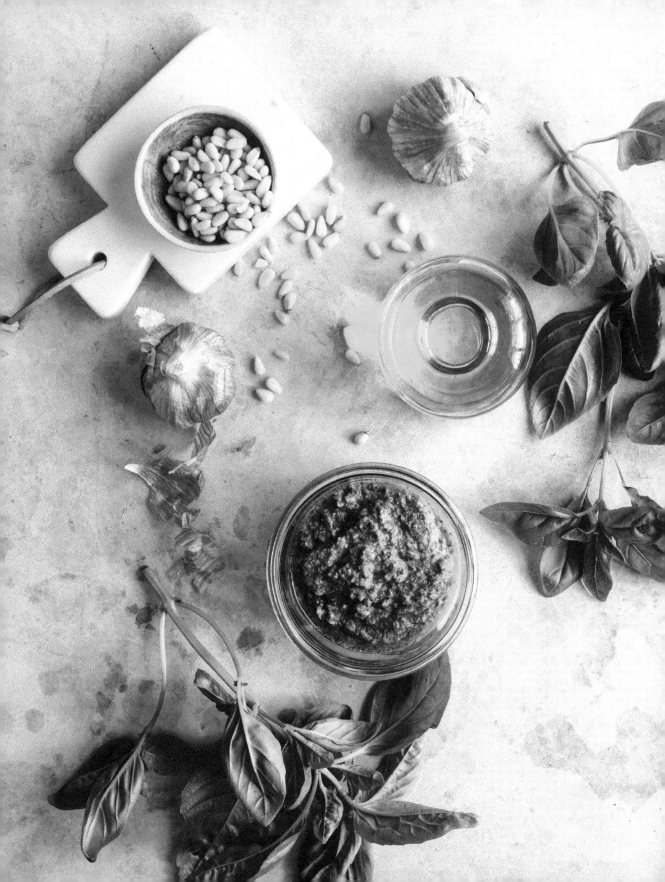

8

Staples

Vegetable Broth

MAKES 8 CUPS (3G CARBS PER SERVING)

Homemade vegetable broth is cheap, easy to make, and tastes so much better (and less salty) than store-bought. Use any vegetables and herbs you like, but make sure to include some aromatics like onions, celery, and carrots. (Stay away from leafy greens and strong-smelling vegetables like turnips.) I keep a bag of veggie scraps like broccoli stems in my freezer and pull it out when I'm ready to make broth.

2 or 3 (4-inch) rosemary sprigs

2 or 3 (4-inch) thyme sprigs

2 or 3 (4-inch) parsley sprigs

1 large onion (unpeeled), root end trimmed, quartered

2 large carrots (unpeeled), washed, ends trimmed, and each cut into 4 pieces

2 celery stalks (including leaves), ends trimmed and each cut into 4 pieces

4 garlic cloves, peeled and left whole

2 bay leaves

½ teaspoon peppercorns

1. Using kitchen twine, tie together the rosemary, thyme, and parsley. (If you don't have twine, don't worry about it. Tying the herbs together just makes it easier to discard them later.)

2. In the electric pressure cooker, combine the onion, carrots, celery, garlic, bay leaves, and peppercorns. Drop the herb bundle on top, then pour in 6 cups of water.

3. Close and lock the lid of the pressure cooker. Set the valve to sealing.

4. Cook on high pressure for 15 minutes.

5. When the cooking is complete, hit Cancel. Allow the pressure to release naturally for 15 minutes, then quick release any remaining pressure.

6. Once the pin drops, unlock and remove the lid.

7. Cool the broth to room temperature, then strain it through a fine-mesh strainer lined with cheesecloth. Discard the solids.

8. Transfer to storage containers and refrigerate for 3 to 4 days or freeze for up to 1 year.

Repurpose tip: Freeze the broth in whatever serving size makes sense for you, and use it whenever a recipe calls for vegetable broth. I like to freeze some 2-cup portions and some 4-cup portions.

Chicken Bone Broth

MAKES 8 CUPS (3G CARBS PER SERVING)

It may seem odd to include vinegar in a recipe for chicken broth, but it's said to help pull nutritious minerals out of the bones, and breaks them down more completely. Leave the skins on your onions for a darker-colored broth. Don't throw out your turkey carcass after Thanksgiving—break up the bones and make turkey bone broth.

2 or 3 (4-inch) rosemary sprigs

2 or 3 (4-inch) thyme sprigs

2 or 3 (4-inch) parsley sprigs

Bones from a 3- to 4-pound chicken

1 large onion (unpeeled), root end trimmed, quartered

2 large carrots (unpeeled), washed, ends trimmed, and each cut into 4 pieces

2 celery stalks (including leaves), ends trimmed and each cut into 4 pieces

2 bay leaves

⅛ teaspoon black peppercorns

1 teaspoon kosher salt (optional)

1 tablespoon apple cider vinegar

1. Using kitchen twine, tie together the rosemary, thyme, and parsley. (If you don't have any twine, don't worry about it. Tying the herbs together just makes it easier to discard them later.)

2. In the electric pressure cooker, combine the bones, onion, carrots, celery, bay leaves, peppercorns, and salt (if using). Drop the herb bundle on top, then add the vinegar and 8 cups of water.

3. Close and lock the lid of the pressure cooker. Set the valve to sealing.

4. Cook on high pressure for 2 hours.

5. When the cooking is complete, hit Cancel. Allow the pressure to release naturally for 20 minutes, then quick release any remaining pressure.

6. Once the pin drops, unlock and remove the lid.

7. Cool the broth to room temperature, then strain it through a fine-mesh strainer lined with cheesecloth. Discard the solids.

8. Transfer to storage containers and refrigerate for 3 to 4 days, or freeze for up to 1 year.

Ingredient tip: Stock and bone broth are essentially the same thing, made by simmering bones for a long period of time to let the collagen seep out. Broth is generally thinner and gets its flavor from meat rather than bones.

PREP TIME:
11 minutes

COOK SETTING:
High

PRESSURE-UP TIME: 24 minutes

COOK TIME:
2 hours

RELEASE: Natural for 20 minutes, then Quick

TOTAL TIME:
2 hours 57 minutes

SPECIAL EQUIPMENT:
fine-mesh strainer, cheesecloth

20-MINUTES-OR-LESS PREP

GLUTEN FREE

LOW CARB

SUGAR FREE

FAMILY FRIENDLY

LOW SODIUM

PER SERVING (1 CUP): Calories: 40; Total Fat: 1g; Protein: 6g; Carbohydrates: 3g; Sugars: 0.5g; Fiber: 1g; Sodium: 20mg

Garam Masala

MAKES ⅓ CUP (6G CARBS PER SERVING)

PREP TIME:
5 minutes

TOTAL TIME:
5 minutes

20-MINUTES-OR-LESS PREP

GLUTEN FREE

VEGAN

LOW CARB

SUGAR FREE

FAMILY FRIENDLY

LOW SODIUM

**PER SERVING
(1½ TABLESPOONS):**
Calories: 32;
Total Fat: 1g; Protein: 1g;
Carbohydrates: 6g;
Sugars: 0g; Fiber: 3g;
Sodium: 7mg

Garam masala, a spice blend used in Indian cooking, translates as "hot mixture of spices." There is no one true blend; the combination of spices varies region to region and cook to cook.

2 tablespoons ground cumin

1 tablespoon freshly ground
black pepper

1 tablespoon ground cardamom

1 tablespoon ground coriander

2 teaspoons ground cinnamon

1 teaspoon ground nutmeg

1 teaspoon ground cloves

⅛ teaspoon cayenne pepper
(optional)

In an old spice jar or small bowl, combine the cumin, black pepper, cardamom, coriander, cinnamon, nutmeg, cloves, and cayenne (if using). Mix well and store, covered and in a cool, dry location, for up to 6 months.

Ingredient tip: If you have trouble finding garam masala, make your own simple version using ground spices. For more authentic flavors, roast whole spices in a dry pan, then grind them together in a coffee grinder. To try this, you'll need cumin seeds, peppercorns, cardamom pods (seeds removed), coriander seeds, a cinnamon stick (broken into smaller pieces), whole cloves, and a dried red chile. Grate fresh nutmeg over the mixture after grinding.

5-Minute Pesto

MAKES 1 CUP (1G CARBS PER SERVING)

Pesto adds zest to so many dishes and is great to make in the summer when fresh basil is abundant. Serve it atop 15-Bean Pistou Soup (page 67), swirled into zucchini noodles, smeared onto grilled vegetables, or mixed into chicken salad. Add some pesto to the sauce the next time you make a cauliflower crust pizza.

PREP TIME:
5 minutes

TOTAL TIME:
5 minutes

SPECIAL EQUIPMENT:
food processor

20-MINUTES-OR-LESS PREP

GLUTEN FREE

LOW CARB

SUGAR FREE

FAMILY FRIENDLY

LOW SODIUM

PER SERVING (1 TABLESPOON):
Calories: 94;
Total Fat: 10g; Protein: 2g;
Carbohydrates: 1g;
Sugars: 0g; Fiber: 0g;
Sodium: 71mg

3 garlic cloves, peeled

2 cups packed fresh basil leaves

½ cup freshly grated
   Parmesan cheese

⅓ cup pine nuts

½ cup extra-virgin olive oil

Kosher salt

Freshly ground black pepper

1. With the motor running, drop the garlic cloves through the feed tube of a food processor fitted with the steel blade. Stop the motor, then add the basil, Parmesan, and pine nuts. Pulse a few times until the pine nuts are finely minced.

2. With the motor running, add the olive oil in a steady stream and process until the pesto is completely puréed. Season with salt and pepper.

3. Store, covered, in the refrigerator for up to 2 weeks.

Substitution tip: This recipe will work with lots of different combinations of herbs/greens and nuts. Try mint and parsley with walnuts, or Swiss chard with almonds.

PREP TIME:
1 minute

COOK TIME:
5 to 10 minutes

TOTAL TIME: 6 to
11 minutes

20-MINUTES-OR-
LESS PREP

GLUTEN FREE

VEGAN

LOW CARB

SUGAR FREE

FAMILY FRIENDLY

LOW SODIUM

**PER SERVING
(1 TABLESPOON):**
Calories: 40;
Total Fat: 3g; Protein: 1g;
Carbohydrates: 2g;
Sugars: 0g; Fiber: 1g;
Sodium: 0mg

Toasted Nuts

MAKES ½ CUP (2G CARBS PER SERVING)

Toasted nuts add great crunch and healthy fat to dishes like salads and lettuce wraps. This recipe can be used for whole or chopped walnuts or pecans, shelled pistachios, sliced or slivered almonds, cashews, or just about any other nut you have in the pantry. Just remember: the smaller the pieces, the faster the toasting process will go. Keep an eye especially on sliced or slivered almonds, as it's very easy to over-toast them.

½ cup nuts

1. Heat a dry nonstick pan over medium-high heat.
2. Place the nuts in the pan and toss or stir frequently for 2 to 5 minutes, until they are toasted and fragrant.
3. Remove from the heat and let cool.

Make-ahead tip: Make a big batch of toasted nuts and store them in a covered glass jar or zip-top bag for up to 3 days so you can have them at a moment's notice all week.

Roasted Tomatillo Salsa

MAKES 1 CUP (4G CARBS PER SERVING)

Here's a tart, green alternative to tomato-based salsa that works well in 4-Ingredient Carnitas Posole (page 45), Chicken Salsa Verde with Pumpkin (page 74), and Pork Carnitas (page 94). Use an angled baby spoon to make seeding the serrano chiles easier. If you're watching sodium, reduce the amount of kosher salt.

1 pound tomatillos (about 6 large), papery husks removed, rinsed

½ large onion, quartered

3 serrano chiles, halved lengthwise, seeded

1 tablespoon extra-virgin olive oil

1 teaspoon kosher salt

1 cup (loosely packed) fresh cilantro leaves

1. Preheat the oven to 375°F.
2. In an 8-inch square baking dish, combine the tomatillos, onion, chiles, oil, and salt. Roast for 1 hour or until the vegetables are very soft. Remove from the oven and let cool slightly.
3. Transfer everything from the baking dish to a food processor, and add the cilantro. Purée until almost smooth. Pour the salsa into a glass jar and store, covered, in the refrigerator for up to 1 week.

Ingredient tip: Tomatillos (pronounced "toe-mah-TEE-yos") look like green tomatoes wrapped in paper-thin husks. To use them, you remove the husks and then rinse off the sticky substance from the skin. Tomatillos are quite tart and can be eaten raw or cooked. They are one of the ingredients in Moroccan Eggplant Stew (page 52).

PREP TIME:
5 minutes

COOK TIME:
1 hour

TOTAL TIME:
1 hour 5 minutes

SPECIAL EQUIPMENT:
food processor

20-MINUTES-OR-LESS PREP

GLUTEN FREE

VEGAN

LOW CARB

FAMILY FRIENDLY

PER SERVING (2 TABLESPOONS):
Calories: 33;
Total Fat: 2g; Protein: 1g;
Carbohydrates: 4g;
Sugars: 2g; Fiber: 1g;
Sodium: 187mg

PREP TIME:
10 minutes

TOTAL TIME:
10 minutes

SPECIAL
EQUIPMENT:
food processor

20-MINUTES-OR-
LESS PREP

GLUTEN FREE

VEGAN

LOW CARB

FAMILY FRIENDLY

LOW SODIUM

PER SERVING
(2 TABLESPOONS):
Calories: 7;
Total Fat: 0g; Protein: 0g;
Carbohydrates: 2g;
Sugars: 1g; Fiber: 1g;
Sodium: 2mg

Low-Sodium Salsa

MAKES 1 CUP (2G CARBS PER SERVING)

After my best friend had a heart attack, she went on a salt-restricted diet. It surprised her to learn that most bottled salsas contain ridiculous amounts of sodium. Some contain unnecessary sugar, too. Make your own salsa from fresh ingredients, and you won't need to worry about either.

8 ounces cocktail tomatoes, quartered

2 scallions, white and light green parts only, chopped

1 jalapeño chile, seeded and chopped

2 tablespoons chopped fresh cilantro

1 tablespoon freshly squeezed lime juice

1. In a food processor, combine the tomatoes, scallions, jalapeño, cilantro, and lime juice. Pulse until the salsa is the consistency you like. If you don't have a food processor, finely chop the tomatoes, scallions, and jalapeño, then mix with the cilantro and lime juice.

2. Store, covered, in the refrigerator for up to 3 days.

Substitution tip: This recipe can easily be customized. If you can't find cocktail tomatoes, use regular tomatoes or cherry tomatoes. If you don't have any scallions, use about a tablespoon of chopped red or yellow onion instead. If you aren't a fan of spicy food, try green bell pepper in place of the jalapeño. If you're a true chile-head, add some chopped habanero. (Make sure to use gloves when you chop hot peppers!)

Spiced Tomato Ketchup

MAKES 4 CUPS (5G CARBS PER SERVING)

Have you ever thought about making your own ketchup? It's easy, and you can spice it however you want. My husband likes to drizzle this ketchup over Lentils with Carrots (page 61) and Curried Black-Eyed Peas (page 63). I like it with baked sweet potato fries. The ketchup will keep, covered, in the refrigerator for up to two months, but a sauce this tasty may not be around that long.

1 (28-ounce) carton or can crushed tomatoes

1 (6-ounce) can tomato paste

½ cup finely chopped onion

½ cup cider vinegar

¼ cup pure maple syrup

½ teaspoon dry mustard (such as Colman's)

¼ teaspoon ground allspice

¼ teaspoon ground cinnamon

¼ teaspoon ground mace

¼ teaspoon ground ginger

¼ teaspoon ground cloves

¼ teaspoon red pepper flakes (optional)

¼ teaspoon kosher salt

Freshly ground black pepper

1. In the electric pressure cooker, combine the tomatoes, tomato paste, onion, vinegar, maple syrup, mustard, allspice, cinnamon, mace, ginger, cloves, red pepper flakes (if using), salt, and pepper. Stir well.

2. Close and lock the lid of the pressure cooker. Set the valve to sealing.

3. Cook on high pressure for 15 minutes.

4. When the cooking is complete, hit Cancel. Allow the pressure to release naturally for 10 minutes, then quick release any remaining pressure.

5. Once the pin drops, unlock and remove the lid.

6. Use an immersion blender right in the pot to get the ketchup to a nice, thick consistency. If it looks watery at all, hit Sauté and let the ketchup simmer until it is the correct thickness. It should fall off of a spoon while slightly resisting.

7. Let the ketchup cool to room temperature, then store it, covered, in the refrigerator for up to 2 months.

Substitution tip: If you don't feel like measuring all of the spices, replace the allspice, cinnamon, mace, ginger, and cloves with 1¼ teaspoons of pumpkin pie spice or apple pie spice.

PREP TIME:
10 minutes

COOK SETTING:
High

PRESSURE-UP TIME: 12 minutes

COOK TIME:
15 minutes

RELEASE: Natural for 10 minutes, then Quick

TOTAL TIME:
47 minutes

SPECIAL EQUIPMENT:
immersion blender

20-MINUTES-OR-LESS PREP

GLUTEN FREE

VEGAN

LOW CARB

FAMILY FRIENDLY

LOW SODIUM

PER SERVING (2 TABLESPOONS):
Calories: 21;
Total Fat: 0g; Protein: 1g;
Carbohydrates: 5g;
Sugars: 3g; Fiber: 1g;
Sodium: 90mg

Marinara Sauce with Red Lentils

SERVES 12 (16G CARBS PER SERVING)

PREP TIME:
15 minutes

COOK SETTINGS:
Sauté, High

SAUTÉ TIME:
10 minutes

**PRESSURE-UP
TIME:** 12 minutes

COOK TIME:
13 minutes

RELEASE: Natural

TOTAL TIME:
1 hour 12 minutes

**20-MINUTES-OR-
LESS PREP**

GLUTEN FREE

VEGAN

FAMILY FRIENDLY

PER SERVING
(½ **CUP**): Calories: 98;
Total Fat: 3g; Protein: 4g;
Carbohydrates: 16g;
Sugars: 6g; Fiber: 6g;
Sodium: 225mg

This vegan marinara is a great alternative to meat-based sauces. Try it on top of Spaghetti Squash (page 36) or zucchini noodles. Toss it with vegetables and chunks of mozzarella, and stuff the mixture into baked acorn squash. Use it as a sauce for a cauliflower crust pizza. If you like things spicy, add some red pepper flakes or replace the green bell pepper with a hotter variety.

½ cup red lentils

2 tablespoons avocado oil

1 medium onion, chopped

1 small green bell pepper, chopped

1 cup Vegetable Broth (page 116) or low-sodium store-bought vegetable broth

2 tablespoons tomato paste

1 (28-ounce) carton or can crushed tomatoes

1 (14.5-ounce) carton or can diced fire-roasted tomatoes

1 bay leaf

1 tablespoon Italian seasoning

1 teaspoon garlic powder

1 teaspoon brown sugar

Kosher salt

Freshly ground black pepper

1. Pick over the lentils and remove any stones or shriveled lentils. Rinse the lentils in a fine-mesh strainer and drain well.

2. Set the electric pressure cooker to the Sauté setting. When the pot is hot, pour in the avocado oil.

3. Add the onion and green pepper to the pot and sauté for 3 to 5 minutes or until the vegetables begin to soften. Hit Cancel.

4. Add the broth to the pot and scrape up any brown bits. Stir in the tomato paste.

5. Add the lentils, crushed tomatoes, diced tomatoes and their juices, bay leaf, Italian seasoning, garlic powder, and brown sugar. Stir well.

6. Close and lock the lid. Turn the pressure valve to sealing.

7. Cook on high pressure for 13 minutes.

8. When the cooking is complete, hit Cancel. Allow the pressure to release naturally.

9. Once the pin drops, unlock and remove the lid.

10. Season with salt and pepper and stir well.

11. If the sauce is too thin for your liking, you can either use an immersion blender to blend it to the desired consistency or turn the pot back to Sauté/Less and cook for 5 to 10 minutes, stirring occasionally, until the sauce thickens.

Ingredient tip: Lentils come in many different varieties. Red lentils tend to be more delicate than green or brown ones, and they pretty much disintegrate when cooked. This makes them perfect for thickening sauces, soups, and stews.

Italian Turkey Sausage Meatballs

MAKES ABOUT 24 MEATBALLS (12G CARBS PER SERVING)

PREP TIME:
15 minutes

COOK TIME:
20 to 30 minutes

TOTAL TIME: 35 to
45 minutes

**20-MINUTES-OR-
LESS PREP**

FAMILY FRIENDLY

**PER SERVING
(4 MEATBALLS):**
Calories: 269;
Total Fat: 13g; Protein: 25g;
Carbohydrates: 12g;
Sugars: 3g; Fiber: 1g;
Sodium: 877mg

I love Ina Garten's Italian Wedding Soup. These meatballs are similar to the ones she uses in the soup, but bigger and rounder. I make a batch or two and keep them in the freeze   an make either the soup or Spaghetti and Turkey Meatballs   snap. The meatballs are also great   es and pasta sauce.

½ cup freshly grated
   Parmesan cheese

t or

3 tablespoons nonfat milk

1 large egg, lightly beaten

1 teaspoon kosher salt

sley

½ teaspoon freshly ground
   black pepper

cken, sausage, breadcrumbs, garlic, parsley, Parmesan, milk, egg, salt, and pepper. Mix gently but thoroughly. (I like to use my hands.)

3. Line a sheet pan with parchment paper. Pinch off about 1 tablespoon of the meat mixture and roll it into a ball. A 1¼-inch cookie scoop makes the job easy. Place the meatball on the sheet pan and repeat with the remaining meat. You should end up with about 24 meatballs.

4. If you plan to eat the meatballs right away, bake them for 30 minutes or until they are lightly browned and cooked through. If you plan to freeze the meatballs, bake them for 20 minutes, then let them cool before freezing.

Substitution tip: Use ground chicken or ground turkey with either Italian-style turkey or chicken sausage. You can go all chicken or all turkey, if desired, but I like to use a combination of the two. Make sure your sausage is not precooked.

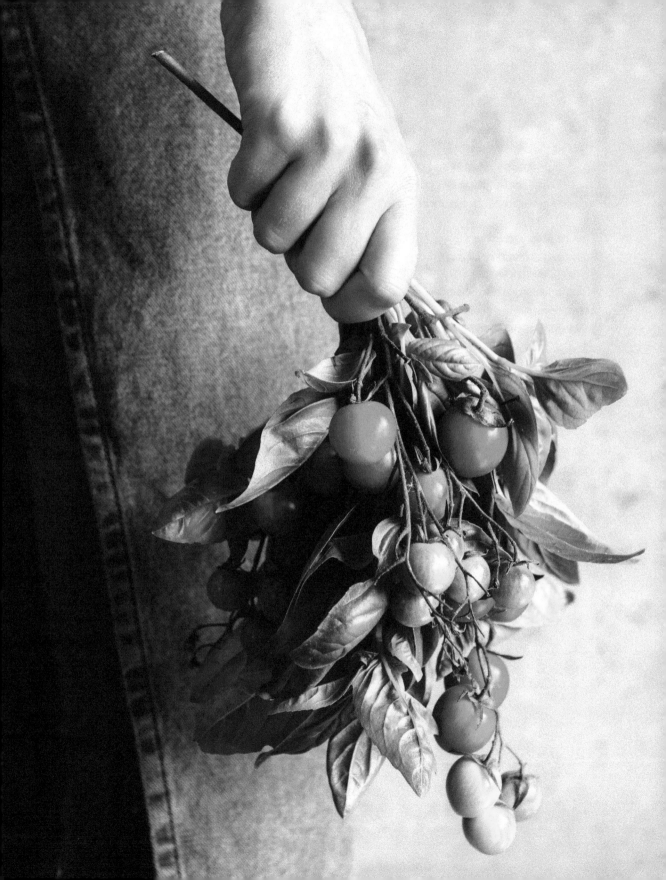

Measurement Conversions

VOLUME EQUIVALENTS (LIQUID)

US STANDARD	US STANDARD (OUNCES)	METRIC (APPROXIMATE)
2 tablespoons	1 fl. oz.	30 mL
¼ cup	2 fl. oz.	60 mL
½ cup	4 fl. oz.	120 mL
1 cup	8 fl. oz.	240 mL
1½ cups	12 fl. oz.	355 mL
2 cups or 1 pint	16 fl. oz.	475 mL
4 cups or 1 quart	32 fl. oz.	1 L
1 gallon	128 fl. oz.	4 L

OVEN TEMPERATURES

FAHRENHEIT	CELSIUS (APPROXIMATE)
250°F	120°C
300°F	150°C
325°F	165°C
350°F	180°C
375°F	190°C
400°F	200°C
425°F	220°C
450°F	230°C

VOLUME EQUIVALENTS (DRY)

US STANDARD	METRIC (APPROXIMATE)
⅛ teaspoon	0.5 mL
¼ teaspoon	1 mL
½ teaspoon	2 mL
¾ teaspoon	4 mL
1 teaspoon	5 mL
1 tablespoon	15 mL
¼ cup	59 mL
⅓ cup	79 mL
½ cup	118 mL
⅔ cup	156 mL
¾ cup	177 mL
1 cup	235 mL
2 cups or 1 pint	475 mL
3 cups	700 mL
4 cups or 1 quart	1 L

WEIGHT EQUIVALENTS

US STANDARD	METRIC (APPROXIMATE)
½ ounce	15 g
1 ounce	30 g
2 ounces	60 g
4 ounces	115 g
8 ounces	225 g
12 ounces	340 g
16 ounces or 1 pound	455 g

The Dirty Dozen and the Clean Fifteen™

A nonprofit environmental watchdog organization called Environmental Working Group (EWG) looks at data supplied by the US Department of Agriculture (USDA) and the Food and Drug Administration (FDA) about pesticide residues. Each year it compiles a list of the best and worst pesticide loads found in commercial crops. You can use these lists to decide which fruits and vegetables to buy organic to minimize your exposure to pesticides and which produce is considered safe enough to buy conventionally. This does not mean they are pesticide-free, though, so wash these fruits and vegetables thoroughly.

DIRTY DOZEN™

apples
celery
cherries
grapes
nectarines
peaches

pears
potatoes
spinach
strawberries
sweet bell peppers
tomatoes

Additionally, nearly three-quarters of hot pepper samples contained pesticide residues

CLEAN FIFTEEN™

asparagus
avocados
broccoli
cabbages
cantaloupes

cauliflower
eggplants
honeydew melons
kiwis
mangoes

onions
papayas
pineapples
sweet corn
sweet peas (frozen)

Cooking Charts

The following charts provide approximate cook times used for a variety of foods in a 6-quart electric pressure cooker like the Instant Pot. Larger electric pressure cookers may need a little extra time to cook. To begin, you may want to cook for a minute or two less than the times listed; you can always simmer foods at natural pressure to finish cooking.

Keep in mind that these times apply to the foods when partially submerged in water (or broth), steamed, or cooked alone. However, the cooking times for a given food may differ when it's used in different recipes, because of additional ingredients or cooking liquids, a different release method than the one listed here, and so on.

For any foods labeled "natural release," allow at least 15 minutes of natural pressure release before quick releasing any remaining pressure.

Beans and Legumes

When cooking a pound or more of beans, it's best to use low pressure and increase the cooking time by a minute or two, because larger amounts at high pressure are prone to foaming. If you have less than a pound of beans, high pressure is fine. A little oil in the cooking liquid will reduce foaming as well.

Unless a shorter release time is indicated, let the pressure release naturally for at least 15 minutes, after which any remaining pressure can be quick released.

	MINUTES UNDER PRESSURE UNSOAKED	MINUTES UNDER PRESSURE SOAKED IN SALTED WATER	PRESSURE	RELEASE
Black beans	22 25	10 12	High Low	Natural
Black-eyed peas	12 15	5 7	High Low	Natural for 8 minutes, then quick
Cannellini beans	25 28	8 10	High Low	Natural
Chickpeas (garbanzo beans)	18 20	3 4	High Low	Natural for 3 minutes, then quick
Kidney beans	25 28	8 10	High Low	Natural
Lentils	10	Not recommended	High	Quick
Lima beans	15 18	4 5	High Low	Natural for 5 minutes, then quick
Navy beans	18 20	8 10	High Low	Natural
Pinto beans	25 28	10 12	High Low	Natural
Soybeans, dried	25 28	12 14	High Low	Natural
Soybeans, fresh (edamame)	1	Not recommended	High	Quick
Split peas (unsoaked)	5 (firm peas) to 8 (soft peas)	Not recommended	High	Natural

Grains

To prevent foaming, it's best to rinse grains thoroughly before cooking, or include a small amount of butter or oil with the cooking liquid. Unless a shorter release time is indicated, let the pressure release naturally for at least 15 minutes, after which any remaining pressure can be quick released.

	LIQUID PER 1 CUP OF GRAIN	MINUTES UNDER PRESSURE	PRESSURE	RELEASE
Arborio (or other medium-grain) rice	1½ cups	6	High	Quick
Barley, pearled	2½ cups	10	High	Natural
Brown rice, long grain	1½ cups	13	High	Natural for 10 minutes, then quick
Brown rice, medium grain	1½ cups	6–8	High	Natural
Buckwheat	1¾ cups	2–4	High	Natural
Farro, pearled	2 cups	6–8	High	Natural
Farro, whole grain	3 cups	22–24	High	Natural
Oats, rolled	3 cups	3–4	High	Quick
Oats, steel-cut	4 cups	12	High	Natural
Quinoa	2 cups	2	High	Quick
Wheat berries	2 cups	30	High	Natural for 10 minutes, then quick
White rice, long grain	1½ cups	3	High	Quick
Wild rice	2½ cups	18–20	High	Natural

Meat

Except as noted, the times below are for braised meats—that is, meats that are seared before pressure-cooking and partially submerged in liquid. Unless a shorter release time is indicated, let the pressure release naturally for at least 15 minutes, after which any remaining pressure can be quick released.

	MINUTES UNDER PRESSURE	PRESSURE	RELEASE
Beef, shoulder (chuck), 2" chunks	20	High	Natural for 10 minutes
Beef, shoulder (chuck) roast (2 lb.)	35	High	Natural
Beef, bone-in short ribs	40	High	Natural
Beef, flat iron steak, cut into ½" strips	1	Low	Quick
Beef, sirloin steak, cut into ½" strips	1	Low	Quick
Lamb, shanks	40	High	Natural
Lamb, shoulder, 2" chunks	35	High	Natural
Pork, back ribs (steamed)	30	High	Quick
Pork, shoulder, 2" chunks	20	High	Natural
Pork, shoulder roast (2 lb.)	25	High	Natural
Pork, smoked sausage, ½" slices	20	High	Quick
Pork, spare ribs (steamed)	20	High	Quick
Pork, tenderloin	4	Low	Quick

Poultry

Except as noted, the times below are for poultry that is partially submerged in liquid. Unless a shorter release time is indicated, let the pressure release naturally for at least 15 minutes, after which any remaining pressure can be quick released.

	MINUTES UNDER PRESSURE	PRESSURE	RELEASE
Chicken breast, bone-in (steamed)	8	Low	Natural for 5 minutes
Chicken breast, boneless (steamed)	5	Low	Natural for 8 minutes
Chicken thigh, bone-in	15	High	Natural for 10 minutes
Chicken thigh, boneless	8	High	Natural for 10 minutes
Chicken thigh, boneless, 1"–2" pieces	5	High	Quick
Chicken, whole (seared on all sides)	12–14	Low	Natural for 8 minutes
Duck quarters, bone-in	35	High	Quick
Turkey breast, tenderloin (12 oz.) (steamed)	5	Low	Natural for 8 minutes
Turkey thigh, bone-in	30	High	Natural

Seafood

All times are for steamed fish and shellfish.

	MINUTES UNDER PRESSURE	PRESSURE	RELEASE
Clams	2	High	Quick
Halibut, fresh (1" thick)	3	High	Quick
Large shrimp, frozen	1	Low	Quick
Mussels	1	High	Quick
Salmon, fresh (1" thick)	5	Low	Quick
Tilapia or cod, fresh	1	Low	Quick
Tilapia or cod, frozen	3	Low	Quick

Vegetables

The cooking method for all the following vegetables is steaming; if the vegetables are cooked in liquid, the times may vary. Green vegetables will be crisp-tender; root vegetables will be soft. Unless a shorter release time is indicated, let the pressure release naturally for at least 15 minutes, after which any remaining pressure can be quick released.

	PREP	MINUTES UNDER PRESSURE	PRESSURE	RELEASE
Acorn squash	Halved	9	High	Quick
Artichokes, large	Whole	15	High	Quick
Beets	Quartered if large; halved if small	9	High	Natural
Broccoli	Cut into florets	1	Low	Quick
Brussels sprouts	Halved	2	High	Quick
Butternut squash	Peeled, ½" chunks	8	High	Quick
Cabbage	Sliced	5	High	Quick
Carrots	½"–1" slices	2	High	Quick
Cauliflower	Whole	6	High	Quick
Cauliflower	Cut into florets	1	Low	Quick
Green beans	Cut in half or thirds	1	Low	Quick
Potatoes, large russet (for mashing)	Quartered	8	High	Natural for 8 minutes, then quick
Potatoes, red	Whole if less than 1½" across; halved if larger	4	High	Quick
Spaghetti squash	Halved lengthwise	7	High	Quick
Sweet potatoes	Halved lengthwise	8	High	Natural

Recipe Index

Index

Acknowledgments

Many thanks to Kim Suarez, Elizabeth Castoria, and the rest of the talented team at Callisto Media. Without them, this book would never have come to life.

We'd also like to send a special shout-out to Mary Opfer, Anna Norton, Marilyn Heneghan, and Rick Kinnaird for sharing and testing recipes. Your time and thoughtful comments were truly appreciated.

About the Authors

 Shelby Kinnaird, author of *The Pocket Carbohydrate Counter Guide for Diabetes*, publishes diabetes-friendly recipes and tips for people who want to eat healthy at DiabeticFoodie.com, a website often stamped with a "top diabetes blog" label. She loves food, hence her motto: "A diabetes diagnosis is not a dietary death sentence." Shelby leads two DiabetesSisters support groups in the Richmond, Virginia, area and is a member of the American Diabetes Association's Virginia Advocacy Council. She has successfully managed her type 2 diabetes since 1999.

 Simone Harounian is a registered dietitian and certified diabetes educator. After graduating with a master's degree from New York University, she worked in a clinical setting experiencing multiple facets of the nutrition industry. She found her passion in helping people with diabetes and took her skills from a hospital setting to a private practice. She is an owner of a nutrition consulting business. She has also enjoyed teaching at a local college. Simone loves frequenting farmers' markets, cooking, and traveling to new places. She lives in New York City with her husband, son, and daughter.

CPSIA information can be obtained
at www.ICGtesting.com
Printed in the USA
BVHW051145140219
540185BV00003B/3